Christine Bailey

five weeks to
Gut Health

Easy and Delicious Recipes to Reset, Restore and Replenish your Microbiome

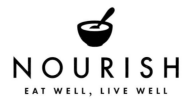

NOURISH

EAT WELL, LIVE WELL

To my three beautiful children, Nathan, Isaac and Simeon, for tasting enthusiastically every recipe created, and to my amazing husband, Chris, for his support and encouragement. Also, to Isaac, who has experienced the healing power of food in resolving his autoimmune condition – you have been my inspiration.

Five Weeks to Gut Health
Christine Bailey

First published in the UK and USA in 2016
This edition published in the UK and USA in 2025 by
Nourish, an imprint of Watkins Media Limited
Unit 11, Shepperton House,
89–93 Shepperton Road
London, N1 3DF

enquiries@nourishbooks.com

Publisher: Fiona Robertson
Commissioning Editor: Sophie Blackman
Managing Editor: Daniel Culver
Designer: Alice Claire Coleman
Commissioned Photography: Toby Scott
Production: Uzma Taj

A CIP record for this book is available from the British Library
ISBN: 978-1-84899-437-9 (paperback)
ISBN: 978-1-84899-438-6 (ebook)
10 9 8 7 6 5 4 3 2 1

Typeset in Brandon Grotesque
Colour reproduction by Rival Colour
Printed in China

Publisher's Note
While every care has been taken in compiling the recipes for this book, Watkins Media Limited, or any other persons who have been involved in working on this publication, cannot accept responsibility for any errors or omissions, inadvertent or not, that may be found in the recipes or text, nor for any problems that may arise as a result of preparing one of these recipes. If you are pregnant or breastfeeding or have any special dietary requirements or medical conditions, it is advisable to consult a medical professional before following any of the recipes contained in this book.

Notes on the Recipes
Some recipes require a high-speed blender or mini food processor for grinding nuts finely.
Unless otherwise stated:
- Use filtered water, if possible, when making fermented foods
- Use organic ingredients and animal products, such as gelatine, from grass-fed animals where possible
- Use medium fruit and vegetables and eggs
- Use fresh ingredients, including herbs and spices
- Do not mix metric and imperial measurements
- 1 tsp = 5ml   1 tbsp = 15ml   1 cup = 250ml

The nutrition information and symbols refer to the recipes only, not including ingredient alternatives, optional ingredients or serving suggestions. Check on the packaging that all ingredients or supplements are vegan, and if required, gluten- and soy-free. Protein powders are considered to be vegan and soy-free (pea, rice or hemp).

nourishbooks.com

FSC
www.fsc.org
MIX
Paper | Supporting
responsible forestry
FSC® C136333

Contents

4	Introduction
5	Understanding Irritable Bowel Syndrome
9	A Closer Look at Your Gut
18	The 5R Approach to a Healthy Happy Gut
27	How to Follow the Programme
32	Five Weeks Using the 5R Approach
37	Basic Recipes
57	Juices, Smoothies & Breakfasts
85	Lunches
113	Main Meals
143	Desserts, Treats & Snacks
174	Notes
179	Index

5-STEP symbols:

REM	Remove
REPL	Replace
REPO	Repopulate
REPA	Repair
REB	Rebalance

DIETARY symbols:

D	Dairy-free
F	Low FODMAP
G	Gluten-free
GR	Grain-free
P	Paleo
S	No added sugar
SC	Specific carbohydrate diet
V	Suitable for vegetarians
VE	Suitable for vegans

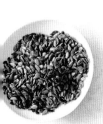
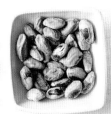
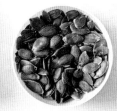
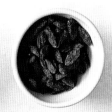

Introduction

If you are struggling with abdominal pain, discomfort, bloating or erratic bowel movements, rest assured you are not alone. Functional bowel disorders (having symptoms without any detectable physical abnormality) such as irritable bowel syndrome (IBS) are very common. In fact, IBS affects about 10 per cent of the global population, and 70 per cent of those suffering are women. For some people, their digestive symptoms are mild, but for many they have a profound effect on their quality of life. They can impact mental and emotional health, sleep, eating patterns and overall feelings of vitality. The aim of this book is to provide information to help you address any potential contributing factors, seek professional support and find practical solutions – through diet and lifestyle – to improve your overall digestive health.

How this book can help you

Functional disorders such as IBS are complex, and there are often no quick fixes. Studies suggest there can be a number of underlying factors and with the right personalized approach it is possible to improve symptoms and overall wellbeing.

Five Weeks to Gut Health will help you understand why your symptoms occur and what you can do to improve them. There is no universal solution, but I have outlined a series of steps for you to follow, based on the 5R approach developed by the Institute of Functional Medicine. The programme encompasses five stages – Reduce/Remove, Replace, Repopulate, Repair and Rebalance (see pages 18–26) – and it aims to help you identify and address any potential imbalances and ultimately improve your overall gut health. It is important to remember that some steps may be more relevant than others, depending on your symptoms, current diet and lifestyle. It is also important to seek professional help (doctor, dietitian, nutritionist) to support you and ensure any appropriate tests or investigations are undertaken.

Understanding Irritable Bowel Syndrome

IBS is the most common digestive disorder. In the UK, for example, it is believed to affect about one in five people. As it is a functional bowel disorder, IBS can be difficult to diagnose and there is no straightforward test that can tell you if you have it. If you think you may have IBS, it is a good idea to see a doctor, instead of trying to figure it out on your own. That way, you can make sure there isn't something else causing your symptoms.

Do I have IBS?

At present IBS is diagnosed based on symptoms defined by the Rome IV Criteria. This system was created by the Rome Foundation, a group of experts in gut health. To be diagnosed with IBS, other conditions must have been ruled out and symptoms must have started at least six months previously. The Rome IV Criteria states you will have recurrent abdominal pain, on average at least one day per week in the past three months, and two or more of the following:

- Pain related to defecation (emptying bowels)
- Pain associated with a change in frequency of stool
- Pain associated with a change in appearance of stool

Interestingly, while bloating is a major complaint for many people with IBS, it is not one of the official criteria.

These are the different types of IBS:

Diarrhoea predominant IBS-D: loose stools more than 25 per cent of the time

Constipation predominant IBS-C: hard stools more than 25 per cent of the time

Mixed or alternating type IBS-M: mixed bowel habits – both hard and soft stools more than 25 per cent of the time

Unspecified IBS-U: bowel habit does not accurately fit any of the above patterns

Act on these red flags

If any of the following additional symptoms or circumstances apply to you, please seek medical advice urgently:

- Very dark stools or blood in the stool
- Unintentional weight loss
- Anaemia
- Family history of ovarian or colon cancer
- Noticeable sudden change in your symptoms
- Symptoms begin after the age of 50

What happens in the gut doesn't stay in the gut!

Many people with IBS deal with more than just tummy troubles. They often feel tired, get backaches, headaches and nausea, or have urinary issues such as needing to go to the toilet all the time or not feeling like they have completely emptied their bladder. In addition, IBS symptoms can overlap with those of other conditions. It is not unusual for people with IBS to also have disorders like fibromyalgia, chronic fatigue, acid reflux and gastritis (inflammation of the stomach lining). Mental health issues such as depression and anxiety are common in people with IBS, too. This is why fixing your gut can have lasting benefits for your overall health and wellbeing.

Figuring out the causes

Understanding what is causing your digestive issues can really help you manage them better. Things that can mess with your gut health include an imbalanced gut microbiome (the diverse community of microorganisms, such as bacteria, viruses, fungi and other microbes, that inhabit the digestive tract, particularly the large intestine), dietary habits, stress and gut infections. Looking at each area separately can help you find out what is triggering your symptoms, and then work out what to do. Here are some factors to consider.

Trauma during early childhood, such as family conflicts, illness, bereavement or any kind of abuse, can increase the chances of developing IBS later in life.

Stress plays a big role in digestive problems. It affects the gut–brain connection, causing symptoms such as stomach pain and changes in bowel movements. Stress can make existing symptoms worse and/or may contribute to their onset in the first place.

Ever had a nasty case of **traveller's diarrhoea** or **food poisoning**? Unfortunately, these infections can sometimes trigger IBS. They are usually short-lived, but it is a good idea to get a stool test to check for parasitic infections such as Giardia, which has been linked to IBS symptoms. Also, you may be at a higher risk of developing IBS immediately after a bout of food poisoning. This is because such infections can cause low-grade inflammation and increased intestinal permeability (leaky gut; see page 7), which can lead to IBS.[1]

Visceral hypersensitivity is when the nerves in your gut are extra sensitive to stimuli, making you feel pain more easily. It is now clear that people with IBS often have this condition. The heightened sensitivity can affect how urgent your bowel movements feel and can cause abdominal pain. It may even be linked to pain outside of the digestive tract, such as in your joints and back. There seems to be a connection between visceral hypersensitivity and inflammation in IBS, so tackling inflammation may help reduce your abdominal pain and digestive issues. It may be helpful to identify and address factors such as food sensitivity, gut imbalance, diet, stress and so on that could be fuelling an inflammatory response.

Mast cells (part of the immune system) may also play a role in the pain response, releasing histamine (see page 15) and other substances that can make nearby nerve fibres more sensitive. This may explain why some people find that high histamine levels worsen their digestive symptoms.

How healthy is your gut microbiome?

Research shows that people with IBS often have less diverse gut microbes[2] compared to those without digestive issues. This lack of diversity is associated with imbalances in the gut microbiome known as "dysbiosis", which can impact your whole digestive system. In addition, there are usually more pro-inflammatory bacteria and fewer beneficial ones in the gut microbiomes of people with IBS.

When your gut bacteria are out of balance, it can affect your bowel function. In a healthy gut, certain bacteria break down carbohydrates to produce short-chain fatty acids (SCFAs), which are essential for keeping your colon healthy. Dysbiosis can impact the production of these SCFAs,[3] compromising your gut lining's integrity and function. It can also trigger an overactive immune response, leading to inflammation that can disrupt normal gut movement (how quickly food moves through your digestive system) and function. In addition dysbiosis affects the gut-brain axis (see page 8), influencing bowel motility and sensitivity.

There are other imbalances in our gut bacteria such as SIBO (small intestinal bacterial overgrowth), which occurs when there is too much bacteria in the small intestine. SIBO is fairly common in people with IBS,[4] affecting approximately 30 to 50 per cent. It can cause fermentation and malabsorption (difficulty digesting or absorbing nutrients from food), leading to bloating, distention, abdominal pain and changes in bowel habits. For example, methane-producing bacteria can slow down your intestines and cause constipation.[5] Other bacteria can speed things up and cause diarrhoea. Bacterial overgrowth can also lead to fat malabsorption, resulting in fatty stools and deficiencies in fat-soluble vitamins (A, D, E and K). These vitamins are crucial for maintaining gut health and overall wellbeing.[6]

In short, having a diverse range of gut bacteria is crucial for a healthy gut.

What causes the imbalance in our gut bacteria?

Our dietary and lifestyle choices play a pivotal role in dysbiosis.[7] We know, for example, that Western-style diets – rich in saturated fats and sugars, and low in fibre – have been associated with imbalance in our gut bacteria.

Stomach acid is a key defence against microbial infections, and reduced levels of stomach acid (which can occur if you take certain medications, such as proton pump inhibitors to treat acid reflux or stomach ulcers) have been linked to SIBO. Antibiotics can inadvertently deplete our beneficial bacteria, paving the way for less desirable microbes to flourish.

Digestive issues such as ongoing constipation or poor gut motility can lead to food fermenting in our gut, which, in turn, disturbs its microbial balance. Previous gut infections and conditions such as coeliac disease further heighten our susceptibility to dysbiosis.

Addressing bacteria overgrowth and dysbiosis is part of Step 1 Reduce/Remove in the 5R approach (see pages 18–21).

Ever heard of leaky gut?

Often called increased intestinal permeability, leaky gut occurs when the lining of your intestines becomes more permeable than it should be. Normally, this lining acts as a selective barrier, allowing nutrients to pass through while keeping out harmful substances such as bacteria and toxins. It is made up of tightly packed cells held together by junctions that can open and close. Various factors such as diet, stress and the balance of gut bacteria can disrupt these junctions, causing them to become too open. This increased intestinal permeability is associated with conditions such as inflammatory bowel disease (IBD),[8] coeliac disease,[9] autoimmune disorders[10] and IBS.[11]

When the gut becomes leaky, it allows substances like food allergens and bacteria to cross into the bloodstream, triggering inflammation. This inflammation not only affects gut function, but can also influence the gut-brain axis, contributing to symptoms such as chronic pain and sensitivity.[12] Research shows that addressing leaky gut – part of the Repair phase in the 5R programme (see pages 23–24) – plays a crucial role in managing associated conditions and restoring digestive wellness.

What is the gut–brain axis?

The gut–brain axis is like a superhighway of communication between your gut and your brain. Your gastrointestinal tract is lined with its own nervous system, known as the enteric nervous system, and it communicates with the central nervous system through the vagus nerve and spinal cord. This means your emotions, pain and stress can influence how your gut works. They can change how sensitive you are to pain and affect gut movement. Additionally, they play a big role in controlling digestive juices, such as stomach acid and enzymes, which are essential for breaking down food.

The gut–brain axis also involves your immune system. When the immune system in your gut gets activated or there is low-grade inflammation, it can impact both your gut function and brain function.

Importantly, gut–brain communication works both ways. Gut bacteria produce all sorts of metabolites (substances formed or used during metabolism), including SCFAs and neurotransmitters such as serotonin and dopamine, which regulate mood/wellbeing and motivation, respectively. These chemicals can influence pain sensors and pathways, affecting brain function. When the gut microbiome is out of balance, it can mess up the signalling pathways, leading to more inflammation, changes in gut movement and increased gut permeability – all of which can worsen digestive symptoms.

Understanding the gut–brain axis underscores the importance of maintaining balance in your life. This is where Step 5 Rebalance of the 5R approach (see pages 24–26) comes into play. Tackling lifestyle factors such as stress, sleep, mental health and exercise can go a long way to improving your digestive health.

A Closer Look at Your Gut

Your gut microbiota refers to the vast community of microorganisms – bacteria, fungi and viruses – that reside in your digestive tract, primarily in the colon. Each person's microbiota is unique, but having a diverse mix of microorganisms is linked to better overall health. When there is a lack of diversity and/or an imbalance in the gut, this is associated with health issues such as IBD and IBS. Sometimes, bacteria can overgrow in places they shouldn't, like the small intestine, leading to conditions such as SIBO.

Our tiny gut bugs play crucial roles. For example, beneficial bacteria produce SCFAs such as butyrate, which nourishes the cells lining the colon, reduces inflammation and helps lower the risk of colon cancer.[13] Propionate is involved in managing glucose levels and metabolic health,[14] while acetate serves as fuel for other bacteria and may influence appetite.[15]

Beyond digestion, your gut microbiota supports your immune system, helps detoxify harmful substances and prevents the overgrowth of harmful bacteria, yeasts and parasites. It also contributes to the production of essential vitamins such as K and B.

What you eat and how you live significantly impact your gut's microbial community. Including a variety of plant-based foods in your diet – rich in fibre, prebiotics (which feed beneficial bacteria) and polyphenols (which have antioxidant and anti-inflammatory properties) – is beneficial. Fermented foods like yogurt, kefir, miso and sauerkraut can also have positive effects on your microbiota. On the flip side, habits such as smoking and consuming alcohol can disrupt the delicate balance in your gut.

And some diets, including the low FODMAP diet (which limits fermentable carbohydrates; see pages 11–13), may inadvertently reduce healthy bacteria over time. Other factors that influence your gut bugs include some medications, stress and exercise. Interestingly, exercise not only helps manage stress but also supports a healthy gut environment.

If you have IBS, it is essential to monitor how your gut responds to different foods. The long-term goal is to diversify your diet and include a wide range of foods to promote microbiota diversity and enhance your overall health.

How gut bugs influence your skin

Just as our gut influences our brain, our gut microbiota talks to our skin microbiome.[16] Essentially, the health of our skin and gut are interconnected, with microbes and their by-products travelling between the two systems, influencing inflammation and overall health. This means that an imbalance in our gut can send signals to our skin (and vice versa), and recent research has uncovered how imbalances in the gut microbiota can contribute to skin conditions such as eczema, acne and psoriasis.

If you struggle with skin issues, addressing digestive imbalances and promoting a diverse gut microbiota could potentially improve your skin symptoms.

Reactions to food

When it comes to digestive symptoms, many people notice that certain foods make things worse. Some studies show that around 77 per cent of people with IBS react to certain foods.[17] This strong link between food reactions and IBS suggests that what we eat can significantly affect how our gut behaves.

There are several ways in which food can influence digestive symptoms. Problems may be caused by allergies or intolerances, poorly absorbed carbohydrates[18] or not enough fibre.[19] Pinpointing which foods are causing trouble isn't always easy. Some reactions are immediate and obvious, such as a severe allergy that may be life-threatening, but others may show up hours later with symptoms such as itching, hives, nausea or diarrhoea. IgE antibody or skin prick tests can identify allergies, but many food issues aren't that straightforward. (An IgE antibody test measures the amount of immunoglobulin E antibodies in your blood. If you have allergies, your immune system makes more IgE antibodies than normal when exposed to specific allergens.)

Food intolerances are different from allergies. They don't involve your immune system, but can still cause issues like bloating and gas. They happen when your body struggles to digest certain foods, and studies estimate that about 20 per cent of people are affected.[20] If you are intolerant of a certain food, the amount you eat can play a role in how bad your symptoms get, which is why you can sometimes handle a small amount of that food without getting any symptoms.

Navigating food reactions can be tricky, but with the right guidance you can find what works best for your gut health.

Problems with gluten

Coeliac disease is not a food allergy or intolerance but an autoimmune disease. When someone with coeliac disease eats gluten (a protein in wheat, barley and rye), their immune system starts damaging the tiny finger-like villi in the small intestine. These villi are crucial for absorbing nutrients, so as they get damaged the body not only becomes inflamed but also malnourished. About 1 per cent of people have coeliac disease, and its symptoms – tummy pain, constipation, diarrhoea and bloating, for example – overlap with IBS. Fatigue, depression and anxiety are also common in both conditions. Research shows that many people diagnosed with IBS actually have coeliac disease.[21] If you suspect gluten may be causing issues for you, it is, therefore, important to consult your doctor before removing it from your diet. (It is always crucial to get professional advice before cutting out whole food groups.) This will enable the appropriate tests to be carried out. If you do have coeliac disease, you will need to stick to a gluten-free diet for life.

But not everyone who finds gluten problematic has coeliac disease or a wheat allergy. They may have non-coeliac gluten sensitivity (NCGS), which is different. Instead of triggering an autoimmune reaction, NCGS causes gut and other symptoms when gluten is eaten. Studies suggest NCGS may be more common than coeliac disease, possibly affecting 6 to 10 per cent of people.[22] Currently, NCGS is typically diagnosed by ruling out other conditions and seeing if symptoms improve on a gluten-free diet.

Aside from coeliac disease and NCGS, gluten can aggravate IBS and leaky gut in some people.[23] And wheat, barley and rye all contain fructans, a type of FODMAP that can cause digestive symptoms in people who are sensitive to them.

Understanding FODMAPs

FODMAPs are a group of carbohydrates – fermentable oligosaccharides, disaccharides, monosaccharides and polyols – that are not fully digested or absorbed in the small intestine. These carbohydrates can then be fermented by gut bacteria, which may cause issues like gas, bloating and diarrhoea, especially for those with IBS.

Reducing FODMAP foods in the diet has been shown to improve IBS symptoms for some people.[24] Developed by Monash University, this approach involves temporarily cutting out high FODMAP foods to reduce symptoms, then gradually reintroducing them while monitoring for any adverse reactions.

While effective in the short term, following a low FODMAP diet over a long period is not recommended for overall digestive health. The diet restricts many beneficial fermentable fibres, and so can disrupt the gut microbiota and lower the levels of healthy bacteria in the gut, particularly *Bifidobacterium* species. These bacteria are important for producing SCFAs, which help keep the gut happy.

If you decide to try a low FODMAP diet temporarily, it is important to ensure you still consume enough soluble fibre (such as oats, quinoa, chia seeds, flaxseeds, blueberries) to support regular bowel movements. Alternatively, you could focus on reducing specific fermentable carbohydrates that are known to aggravate gut symptoms, such as fructans, lactose (see page 12) and fructose (see page 13). Before you make any changes, it is advisable to seek professional support from a nutritionist or dietitian, for example.

Foods to avoid or select

Examples of high and low FODMAP foods are shown in the table overleaf. For some foods, the quantity eaten in one sitting is important; for example, a small handful of almonds is likely to be fine, but consuming more than 12 almonds in one sitting may result in symptoms. For more details, visit the Monash University website where the diet was developed.[25]

If you wish to follow a low FODMAP diet, select recipes in this book marked with the symbol F, omitting the optional ingredients where necessary. You can also make substitutions to many of the other recipes. Instead of using xylitol or honey, for example, switch to maple syrup. Omit onion and garlic and use only the green tops of spring onions/scallions or chives.

Are fructans a problem for you?

Fructans are found in foods such as wheat, barley, rye, onions, garlic, leeks, beans and pulses. These carbohydrates are not well digested by everyone, especially those with gut issues like IBS.[26]

How much you eat can affect how you feel (which is true for all FODMAPs). Instead of cutting out fructans completely long term, you may find you can handle a small amount. This would be helpful, because fructans are a type of fibre and so bring health benefits, too. Beans and pulses, which contain a range of fermentable fibres (fructans, galacto-oligosaccharides [GOS] and fructose), can be particularly problematic for those with IBS symptoms. You may, however, find a small amount of tinned beans or sprouted beans easier to digest. If you are vegan and concerned about eating sufficient protein, it may be gentler on your gut to choose protein-rich

FOOD TYPE	HIGH FODMAP (REDUCE)	LOW FODMAP (SELECT)
FRUIT	Apples, cherries, pears, plums, dried fruits, mango	Banana, pineapple, papaya, berries, citrus fruits, kiwi fruit, grapes
VEGETABLES	Artichoke, asparagus, beetroot/beet, broccoli, fennel, garlic, leek, mushroom, onion, savoy cabbage	Carrot, celery, chives, courgette/zucchini, green beans, green tops of spring onion/scallion, kale, pepper, pumpkin, spinach, tomato
GRAINS	Gluten-containing grains: wheat, barley, rye	Gluten-free grains: quinoa, rice, millet
BEANS AND PULSES	Lentils, beans (such as kidney, borlotti, cannellini), chickpeas, soybeans	
DAIRY	High-lactose milk products, ice cream, commercial yogurt	Lactose-free products, such as butter, ghee, hard cheese, homemade yogurt and kefir, coconut kefir, almond milk, coconut milk
SWEETENERS	Fructose, honey, xylitol, sorbitol, erythritol, agave nectar	Maple syrup, sucrose, stevia
NUTS AND SEEDS	Cashew nuts, pistachio nuts	Almonds, pumpkin seeds, sunflower seeds, tahini, pecan nuts, walnuts

plant foods, such as tofu, tempeh, natto or pea protein, instead of too many beans and pulses.

Certain recipes have been highlighted as FODMAP friendly throughout this book. If you are following the 5R approach, you may wish to try these recipes during Step 1 Reduce/Remove and monitor whether or not your symptoms ease.

Can you tolerate lactose?

Many people with IBS find their symptoms get worse after having dairy.[27] This is often due to lactose intolerance, where your body cannot fully digest lactose – a natural sugar found in milk and dairy products. Lactose is broken down by the enzyme lactase, but some people do not produce enough of this enzyme. Undigested lactose is then fermented by the gut microbiome, leading to gas, bloating and diarrhoea.

Even if you are lactose intolerant, your tolerance level may vary. The amount eaten will impact whether you experience symptoms. Typically, those with lactose intolerance may be able to tolerate around 12g (0.4oz) lactose per day, which means you do not have to completely eliminate dairy from your diet. Look for lactose-free options or stick to low-lactose foods, such as hard cheese and butter. And if you do have dairy, it may help to spread it out over the day instead of having a lot all at once.

Some people have what is called "secondary lactose intolerance", which is common in undiagnosed coeliac disease or Crohn's disease. This is because the villi in the small intestine (where the lactase enzyme is produced) may be inflamed or damaged. As these underlying conditions are treated and the inflammation or damage to the villi decreases, lactase production can return to normal levels. Consequently, your ability to digest lactose and tolerate dairy products will improve as your small intestine heals and functions more effectively.

As we age, our levels of lactase activity decline and we become more prone to issues with lactose. If you suspect lactose is a problem, seek advice from your doctor.

Does fructose trigger your symptoms?

If you struggle with digestive issues, high levels of fructose in your diet may make things worse. About one in three people with IBS[28] are thought to have fructose intolerance. This happens when your small intestine cannot fully absorb fructose, leading to symptoms such as gas, bloating, cramps and diarrhoea. As with lactose intolerance, everyone's ability to handle fructose varies, and how much you eat at a time matters.

Fructose is found naturally in fruit, fruit juices, agave syrup, honey and some vegetables. It is also found in high-fructose corn syrup, which is used in many processed foods and drinks. The problem is not only how much fructose you eat, but also the ratio of fructose to glucose in your food. When fructose levels are higher than glucose levels, it can trigger symptoms. For example, apples have more fructose than glucose, so they may cause digestive issues for some individuals. Oranges and kiwi fruit have similar amounts of both sugars, and so are less likely to cause a problem.

If you find excess fructose a problem, it doesn't mean you have to give up fruit altogether, but it is wise to think about how much fruit you eat and which types you choose. Monash University offers detailed information on FODMAPs, including fructose levels in various foods.

The problem with polyols

Polyols (which include sorbitol, mannitol, xylitol, maltitol and isomalt) are types of FODMAP found naturally in certain foods, such as apricots, mushrooms and avocado. They are used commercially as sweeteners (xylitol) in products like chewing gum, protein bars and chocolate snacks. Xylitol is a sugar alcohol that looks and tastes like sugar but has fewer calories and doesn't impact blood sugar levels to the same extent as table sugar. You will notice that some of the recipes suggest either caster sugar or xylitol. If you suspect polyols aggravate your symptoms then stick to caster sugar in the recipes.

Other food triggers
Understanding alcohol

If you are dealing with digestive issues, it is important to think about your alcohol intake. Research indicates that alcohol can affect your entire digestive system, from causing heartburn and reflux in the stomach to impacting the small and large intestines. There is also evidence linking alcohol consumption with worsening symptoms of IBS.[29] This is possibly because alcohol can induce changes in the gut microbiota,[30] which can lead to dysbiosis, leaky gut and inflammation.

Certain alcoholic beverages, such as cider (because of its high fructose content) and beer (due to wheat or fructans), may exacerbate gut symptoms. Other types of alcohol, such as wine, are high in histamine, which can further affect your gut health.

If you are experiencing digestive discomfort, consider removing alcohol from your diet for a few weeks to see if your symptoms improve. You can do this as part of Step 1 Reduce/Remove of the 5R approach.

Managing caffeine

For some people, caffeine can worsen existing digestive issues.[31] Caffeine is known to stimulate the gastrointestinal tract, which can lead to increased muscle contractions in the intestines and colon. This may result in symptoms such as abdominal pain, urgency to use the bathroom and diarrhoea. Interestingly, for those dealing with constipation, caffeine may offer relief. It is important to note that the impact of caffeine varies from person to person, and not everyone will experience digestive symptoms.

If you suspect caffeine may be triggering your gut symptoms, try monitoring how you feel after you have consumed caffeinated beverages. Consider reducing your caffeine intake to see if symptoms improve. Switching to decaffeinated options may be a beneficial step toward managing your gut health.

The power of fibre

Fibre does far more than just keep your digestion regular: it plays a crucial role in your overall health. Found in plants, fibre is a type of complex carbohydrate that the body cannot fully digest. Instead, fibre travels to the large intestine where gut microbes break it down. In doing so, they produce beneficial compounds such as the SCFAs butyrate, propionate and acetate, which not only nourish the gut lining, but also support brain health, immune function and metabolism.

If you struggle with IBS, you may be more sensitive to certain types of fibre, particularly insoluble fibres found in wheat, certain wholegrains, legumes and corn. Some fibres can add bulk to stools,[32] which may, in turn, distend the colon and potentially worsen IBS symptoms. Some fibre-rich foods, including wheat cereals and bran, are also high in FODMAPs, which can further aggravate the gut. For managing IBS, the British Society of Gastroenterology advises avoiding insoluble fibre because it may increase bloating and abdominal pain. Soluble fibre (oats, oat bran, flaxseed, chia seeds, sweet potato, apples, bananas, pears, carrots, psyllium husk, for example), on the other hand, can be beneficial.

The current recommendation is to consume 30g (1oz) of fibre daily, but most people fail to reach this amount. When increasing fibre intake, do so gradually to prevent bloating and discomfort. The easiest way to increase your fibre intake is to include a greater variety of plants in your diet. The American Gut Project highlights the benefits of doing this, recommending consuming at least 30 different plant foods weekly, including wholegrains, fruits, vegetables, nuts, seeds, legumes, herbs and spices. As you incorporate more fibre-rich foods, pay attention to how your body responds. Starting with less fermentable (lower FODMAP) fibres such as flaxseed, chia seeds, oats, berries, root vegetables, citrus fruits and kiwi may be easier on your digestion initially. However, for long-term digestive health, aim to include a wide range of plant foods in your diet to enhance the diversity of your gut microbiome.

Histamine and gut symptoms

Histamine is a naturally occurring compound in the body that plays a crucial role in the immune system. It acts as a neurotransmitter and regulates various physiological processes, including digestion, sleep and inflammatory responses. Increasingly, histamine is recognized for its potential to cause digestive issues. Histamine intolerance[33] occurs when your body has an impaired ability to break down histamine in the gut, primarily due to a deficiency in the enzyme diamine oxidase (DAO). This causes histamine to build up, triggering digestive symptoms such as bloating, diarrhoea and abdominal pain, as well as broader symptoms such as headaches, eczema and flushing. Elevated histamine levels in the gut can also trigger inflammation, altering gut function and

contributing to the pain and discomfort typical of IBS. Research suggests that an imbalanced gut microbiome may contribute to histamine intolerance by promoting gut inflammation, reducing DAO enzyme activity and increasing leaky gut.

Foods and drinks that are high in histamine include alcohol (wine, beer, cider), pickled and fermented foods (sauerkraut, kimchi, vinegar, soy sauce, miso, aged cheeses), smoked meats, canned fish, shellfish and yeast products. Other foods can trigger histamine release, such as citrus fruits, tomatoes, bananas, nuts, avocados and strawberries. As such, consuming these foods in large quantities can lead to an increase in histamine levels in the body. This can exacerbate gut symptoms for individuals who are intolerant of histamine.

There is still debate on which foods should be avoided if you are trying to manage histamine intolerance. If you think histamine may be contributing to your gut symptoms, consider reducing high histamine foods or taking a DAO supplement to help break down histamine. Some nutrients, including vitamin C,[34] vitamin B6, quercetin[35] and omega-3 fatty acids (from fish or krill oil, flaxseed oil)[36] may also help lower histamine levels. The quality and age of the food, not just the type of food itself, can affect histamine levels.

Since histamine intolerance varies from person to person, it is important to find out which foods and how much you can tolerate. The aim is to avoid eliminating foods altogether because being overly restrictive can impact your gut microbiome, too.

HIGH HISTAMINE FOODS	HISTAMINE RELEASE FOODS
Fermented foods (sauerkraut, kimchi, miso, kombucha)	Citrus fruits (oranges, lemons, limes)
Aged cheeses (cheddar, Gouda, Parmesan)	Strawberries
Cured meats (salami, ham, sausages)	Pineapple
Alcoholic beverages (wine, beer, champagne)	Tomato
Vinegar-containing foods (pickles, vinegar)	Banana
Smoked and/or canned fish (smoked salmon, mackerel, herring, tuna)	Avocado
Spinach	Spinach
Aubergine/eggplant	Chocolate
Tomato	Nuts (walnuts, cashew, peanuts)
Dried fruits (raisins, apricots)	Certain spices (paprika, chili powder)
Aged or fermented soy products (soy sauce, tempeh, miso)	Wheat germ

Nickel sensitivity and gut symptoms

You may have heard of nickel sensitivity affecting the skin, but recent studies suggest that, for some, it can impact gut symptoms. For those sensitive to nickel, foods high in nickel may worsen symptoms of IBS. Nickel can trigger immune reactions and inflammation in sensitive individuals, leading to abdominal pain, bloating and changes in bowel habits.[37]

Common foods that are high in nickel include

chocolate, nuts, seeds, soybeans, oats, certain grains and various vegetables. Interestingly, stainless steel cookware can also release nickel during cooking, adding to your exposure.[38]

If you suspect nickel sensitivity may be contributing to your digestive symptoms, consider reducing your intake of nickel-rich foods and getting rid of any stainless steel cookware that you use.

Boosting gut health with prebiotics

Prebiotics are a vital part of a healthy diet, alongside dietary fibre. They encompass both fibrous and non-fibrous compounds that are food sources for the beneficial microbes residing in the gut. Although we cannot digest prebiotics ourselves, they are broken down by specific beneficial microbes, such as *Lactobacillus* and *Bifidobacterium* species.

By promoting the growth and activity of these beneficial microbes, prebiotics play a crucial role in supporting our immune system and enhancing our metabolic health. This includes regulating insulin and maintaining healthy lipid levels (such as triglycerides, phospholipids and cholesterol). Additionally, prebiotics aid the production of SCFAs, which, as we know, provide numerous benefits to both our gut and overall body health.

Prebiotics are found in different forms, including prebiotic dietary fibres, resistant starches (oats, green bananas, wholegrains, beans and legumes, for example) and polyphenols (in many fruits, nuts, tea, coffee and chocolate, for example). While some prebiotic-rich foods may be high in FODMAPs (onions and garlic, for example) and may potentially exacerbate gut symptoms in sensitive individuals, there are plenty of others that are more easily tolerated. These include berries, apples, oats, bananas, and cooked and cooled potatoes and rice. Incorporating these prebiotic-rich foods into your everyday diet can help support a healthy gut microbiome and improve your overall digestive wellness.

Understanding probiotics for gut health

Probiotics are foods or supplements that contain live bacteria that can be beneficial for your health. Inside your body, there are approximately 100 trillion bacteria, and research has revealed that the types and amounts of these microorganisms in your gut can either prevent or promote the development of various diseases.

Common probiotics include specific strains of bacteria such as *Lactobacillus* species, *Bifidobacterium* species, *Saccharomyces boulardii* and *Bacillus coagulans*, among many others. These probiotics can be found naturally in certain foods, such as fermented milk products (like plain yogurt and kefir), kombucha, sauerkraut, miso, kimchi, tempeh, natto and certain types of pickles. Incorporating these foods into your diet can help balance your gut microbiota and support a healthy immune response.

Some probiotics may only have a temporary effect and do not permanently colonize the gut, but they still contribute to gut health by creating a favourable environment for a diverse microbiome. This is why fermented foods are included in many of the recipes in this book and play a crucial role in Step 3 Repopulate of the 5R approach (see pages 22–23).

The 5R Approach to a Healthy Happy Gut

This five-step programme is a structured approach to improve overall digestive health. It is based on the 5R framework for restoring gut health devised by the Institute of Functional Medicine.[39] The programme is useful for a range of digestive concerns and associated symptoms. Since the digestive tract is where most of our immune cells are and where we absorb nutrients, it makes sense that improving gut health will support overall wellness.

Encompassing five stages – Reduce/Remove, Replace, Repopulate, Repair and Rebalance – the 5R approach enables you to work on key areas that may be causing or exacerbating digestive issues. It is important that you personalize the programme, and it is likely that some of the stages will be more relevant than others. Having read thus far, you have hopefully already identified potential areas that may need your focus.

While the 5R approach is presented as a series of steps, you can work on multiple phases at the same time. For example, removing foods that irritate your digestive tract in Step 1 may improve symptoms and lower the inflammatory response. However, if you are not tackling poor sleep or stress (Step 5 Rebalance), then you are unlikely to feel the full benefits. For this reason, and as a foundation for good health, I suggest you incorporate strategies to reduce stress, improve sleep and do some daily exercise as soon as you start the programme. Your goal is to improve your gut health and function, and in the long term you want to be able to enjoy a wide range of foods without experiencing symptoms.

Step 1: Reduce/Remove

First, we want to find ways to reduce symptoms such as constipation, diarrhoea and bloating. Second, we want to identify and remove any trigger foods that are aggravating or causing these symptoms. This is where the support of a healthcare practitioner (doctor, dietitian, nutritionist) can be helpful. There may be underlying conditions that need to be ruled out, such as SIBO, coeliac disease and so on. In some cases, laboratory testing and appropriate investigations may be required.

As we know, diet plays a key role in gut health so keeping a record of your symptoms and eating patterns may help identify suspect foods. Track your progress and note when you use any recipes from this book. By following the recipes, especially those marked "REM" (Remove), you will lower your consumption of many common problematic foods, which will likely reduce your symptoms. Remember, in the long term, you don't want to overly restrict your diet by removing foods unnecessarily. Use this first step to identify your specific triggers.

Many of the recipes in this book are relatively low in carbohydrates, which may in itself reduce your symptoms. I have suggested ways to incorporate additional carbohydrates that may be more easily tolerated as you work through the steps. It may take up to 4 weeks for you to notice a difference. As you move through Steps 2 to 5, and your overall digestive function improves, you may be able to start introducing/reintroducing a greater variety of foods and/or larger portions of certain foods to find your tolerance level. How you eat is also important. Eating at regular times, avoiding constant snacking and taking your time to eat may help reduce your symptoms. If you experience constipation, diarrhoea or bloating, consider the general guidelines below.

Food irritants: Eliminate alcohol and reduce caffeine and processed foods. If you suffer with repeated acid reflux, it is important to see a healthcare practitioner to rule out any underlying triggers. You may also want to experiment with removing certain foods, such as chocolate, mint, alcohol, coffee and tea, because these reduce the tone of the sphincter muscle that connects the stomach to the oesophagus, exacerbating reflux symptoms. Other irritants include spicy foods, fried and fatty foods, garlic and onions.

FODMAPs: Some people find temporarily reducing or removing certain FODMAPs beneficial (see pages 11–13). I have listed low FODMAP recipes throughout the book.

Food allergies/intolerances: Consider whether there are any suspect foods. Keep a diary, and try removing these foods from your diet. Monitor your symptoms for signs of improvement before reintroducing the foods.

Medications and supplements: Check any medications or supplements for potential digestive side effects. Speak to your doctor if you are concerned. Even over-the-counter medications (aspirin, ibuprofen and other non-steroidal anti-inflammatory drugs, antacids, for example) may aggravate gut symptoms.

Stress and sleep: Take measures to reduce and manage your daily stress levels, incorporate exercise into your daily routine and pay attention to improving your sleep (Step 5 Rebalance).

Gut dysbiosis and/or gut infections: With the help of a healthcare practitioner, address any bacterial or parasitic infections or dysbiosis that could be impacting your gut health. It may involve taking antibiotic, antiviral or antiparasitic agents from herbal sources, such as oil of oregano or berberine, or pharmaceuticals.

Easing constipation

Constipation can be a major factor in making digestive problems, including IBS, worse. When you are constipated, it means that things move more slowly through your colon. This slow transit time causes more water to be absorbed from the stool, making it harder and more difficult to pass. Hard stools can make your gut more sensitive to pain and discomfort.[40] Constipation can also lead to an imbalance in your gut bacteria, favouring less beneficial types, which may exacerbate IBS symptoms like abdominal pain and bloating.

Since your gut is closely connected to your nervous system, stress and tension can affect gut movement. Mind–body therapies that help manage stress and promote relaxation can improve constipation. Including enough plant-based foods in your diet to get adequate fibre is also crucial. It is best to increase fibre intake gradually and drink plenty of fluids. Here are some foods to help ease constipation.

Kiwi fruit: Consume two kiwi fruits daily. Kiwi fruit is a natural remedy for mild constipation, due to its fibre and water content, and its mild anti-inflammatory and antioxidant properties.[41]

Flaxseed: Adding flaxseed[42] to a meal (for example, sprinkled over porridge, yogurt, soup and so on) can be an effective way to support bowel movements because flaxseed is rich in both soluble and insoluble fibres. Start with 1–2 teaspoons and gradually increase to 1–2 tablespoons. Take flaxseed with plenty of fluids because it absorbs water and so adds bulk to the stool.

Chia seed: Like flaxseed, chia seeds are rich in soluble and insoluble fibres, which help maintain regularity and prevent constipation. The soluble fibre in chia seeds forms a gel-like substance when mixed with water, which helps to soften stools and make them easier to pass. Chia seeds can be added to smoothies or made simply into chia pudding.

Psyllium: Also known as ispaghula, psyllium is a soluble fibre that may help ease constipation. It is readily available as a powder or husk, or in capsule form. It is important to consume sufficient fluid alongside all soluble fibres.

Prunes and apricots: Prunes are commonly known to relieve constipation. Both prunes and apricots contain sorbitol, which can act like a laxative. For some people, though, prunes and apricots may contribute to bloating.

Probiotics: Especially when combined with fibre, probiotics help with constipation by increasing the production of SCFAs, reducing the pH of the colon and increasing bile salt metabolism, all of which help stimulate peristalsis (which moves food through the digestive system). In addition, increasing levels of butyrate by taking butyrate supplements may be useful. Ensure a daily intake of probiotics (fermented foods) and also prebiotic-rich foods such as berries or apple sauce.

If you are struggling with constipation, aim to drink 1.5–2 litres (2.6–3.5 pints) of fluid daily. You may find caffeine (coffee or strong tea) helpful because it can work as a bowel stimulant.

Diarrhoea: Understanding and managing symptoms

If you are dealing with diarrhoea, especially if you have IBS-D, it can be tricky to pinpoint the exact cause. Sometimes, there is no obvious reason. Many people with IBS-D have an imbalance in their gut bacteria, with fewer beneficial strains.

To help manage diarrhoea, you could try probiotic supplements such as *Saccharomyces boulardii* and *Lactobacillus acidophilus*, which have shown positive effects. Including probiotic-rich foods in your diet, such as yogurt, kefir, natto, sauerkraut or kimchi, can also be beneficial. Foods high in pectin, such as apple sauce and green bananas, are known to help ease diarrhoea.[43]

Watch your fibre intake, because sometimes too much fibre can make things worse. Also, caffeine can stimulate bowel movements, so cutting back may help. Pay attention to certain foods that are high in specific FODMAPs (sweeteners such as xylitol and sorbitol, for example) and fruits that are high in fructose. You may also want to look at your consumption of wheat, onions, garlic (high in fructans), dairy (lactose) and alcohol.

For some people, bile acid diarrhoea may be the problem. When your gut has too many bile salts, it can pull more water into the colon, leading to diarrhoea and symptoms such as bloating. Bile acid malabsorption isn't rare, and it can affect up to 30 per cent of people with IBS-D.[44] It may also be linked to other gut issues, including SIBO.[45] It is a good idea to seek professional advice and get the necessary tests to establish whether or not you have this condition. In some cases, bile acid binder medications may be helpful.

Beat the bloat

If you are dealing with bloating, it is important to first rule out underlying conditions such as coeliac disease, SIBO or functional dyspepsia (chronic indigestion). Make sure you are having regular bowel movements – ideally daily.

Here are some things you could do to help.

Watch your FODMAPs: Some carbohydrates can be tough on your gut, especially if they are high in FODMAPs. While fibre is generally good for you, too much can worsen bloating. Opt for low fermentable soluble fibres such as chia seeds and flaxseeds, and avoid wheat products.

Mind your eating habits: Be aware of how certain habits can affect bloating. Constantly chewing gum, eating too quickly and drinking too many carbonated drinks may all contribute to bloating. High-fat meals may also cause bloating, because fatty foods slow down how quickly your stomach empties, thus making you feel fuller for longer. If your bile production or flow is off, it can make fat digestion more difficult and worsen bloating.

Stay active: Regular exercise, especially after meals, can be beneficial. Physical activity helps move gas through your digestive tract and improves gut motility, which can ease bloating.

Try activated charcoal: Some people find that activated charcoal helps with bloating, although research is limited. It may work better when combined with simethicone, a medication that helps reduce gas.[46]

Consider probiotics: Probiotics[47] may also be helpful. Studies have shown that a combination of *Lactobacillus acidophilus* and *Bifidobacterium lactis* Bi-07[48] can be effective. Other research suggests *Bifidobacterium infantis*[49] may provide relief.

Step 2: Replace

This stage of the 5R approach focuses on replacing essential digestive elements and nutrients that may be insufficient. There are various options to consider with regards to taking supplements, and an individualized approach is essential. This may include replacing certain digestive enzymes,[50] lactase[51] or DAO for histamine, or taking bile-supportive supplements. In addition, you may wish to speak with a healthcare practitioner to check for any nutrient insufficiencies, such as B12, iron, calcium, vitamin D, magnesium and zinc, all of which are crucial for overall health and digestion.

Hydrochloric acid in the stomach is critical for digesting protein and activating digestive enzymes. Low levels of hydrochloric acid, known as "hypochlorhydria", can lead to poor digestion and nutrient absorption, particularly of proteins, B12 and iron. Replacing digestive elements by consuming certain foods and drinks may be beneficial for gut health. For example, some foods naturally contain enzymes that help break down food in the gut. These include fresh pineapple (particularly the core), papaya and sprouted seeds. In addition, adding citrus juice or vinegar to a meal can stimulate your digestive secretions. You may also find it beneficial to drink a glass of warm water with the juice of half a lemon at meal times. Ginger tea, bitters[52] (Swedish bitters, gentian root, dandelion bitters, for example) and bitter greens are all known to promote the body's ability to produce digestive substances naturally. Incorporate bitter greens such as rocket/arugula, watercress, spinach, chicory and dandelion leaves into your meals whenever you can.

My versions of traditional recipes for the gut-friendly fermented foods kimchi, sauerkraut and pickles can be found on pages 50–54. Add 1–2 tablespoons of one of these to your meal to stimulate your digestive secretions.

Here are some other ways to help support your digestive function.

Ginger is known for its beneficial effects on digestion due to its ability to stimulate saliva, bile and gastric enzymes.[53] It has been used traditionally to relieve indigestion, vomiting and nausea. Ginger has also been shown to mitigate gastrointestinal symptoms, such as bloating and gas, by enhancing digestive processes and reducing inflammation in the gut.[54]

Artichoke has traditionally been used to support digestive health. There is evidence that artichoke leaves alleviate digestive problems,[55] particularly heartburn and IBS symptoms, by stimulating bile production.

Beetroot/beet, radish (daikon), wasabi and **horseradish** are some other foods thought to stimulate bile flow. All of these feature in recipes in this book.

Zinc plays a crucial role in digestive health, particularly in the production of stomach acid. It is essential for the functioning of gastric mucosa (proper operation of the specialized lining of the stomach) and helps maintain the integrity of the gastrointestinal lining.[56] Make sure you incorporate zinc-rich foods in your daily diet. Examples include seafood, beef, spinach, pork, chicken, pumpkin seeds, cashew nuts, raw cacao, mushrooms and sea vegetables. Many of these feature in recipes in this book.

During Step 2, you also want to try and increase the diversity of plant foods in your diet.

If you have already identified what triggers your symptoms, you should be able to start introducing a wider range of foods. By including many different plant foods, you will ensure a sufficient range of plant fibres to support microbiota diversity and regular bowel movements. As previously mentioned, when it comes to fibre you need to find an amount that works for you, so build up slowly over a number of weeks. As your symptoms improve, try including additional grains as accompaniments to some of the dishes, starting with the lower fermentable grains such as rice, quinoa, buckwheat, amaranth, oats and so on. Think variety and colour on your plate and add an extra vegetable or side salad to each meal.

Step 3: Repopulate

Studies have shown that the gut bacteria of people with coeliac disease, IBS and other digestive symptoms differ from those who have a healthy digestion. Our gut microbiota is particularly sensitive to diet and lifestyle. Changing the type of food you eat, focusing on whole unprocessed foods and reducing sugar and sweeteners can play a key role in re-establishing a healthy microbial population.

During Step 3, it is helpful to introduce fermented vegetables such as kimchi, sauerkraut, pickles and beets, dairy or non-dairy yogurt, and beverages like kefir and kombucha. Try incorporating these into meals or snacks on a daily basis.

To improve the balance of beneficial bacteria in your gut, it may be useful to bolster probiotics with foods that contain prebiotics (to feed probiotic bacteria). Examples include Jerusalem artichoke, berries, apples and pears, banana, cacao, green tea, cruciferous vegetables and fibres such as ground flaxseeds, beans, lentils, chickpeas and globe artichokes. Be mindful that some prebiotics are also high fructan foods – onions, garlic and wheat, for example – which may cause bloating. You can still eat them, but be cautious of the quantity you consume in any one meal.

Step 4: Repair

This step focuses on providing the gut with nutrients that are known to support and repair the delicate mucous membrane of the gut lining and reduce inflammation. It is important to appreciate that your central nervous system directly influences your gastrointestinal function. The way you deal with stress (Step 5 Rebalance) will, therefore, impact healing.

Broth made from meat or poultry bones is rich in gelatine (an easier-to-digest type of collagen), glycine and glucosamine, which are restorative nutrients for the gut lining. The amino acids in bone broth may help support gut lining health.[57] In animal studies of inflammatory bowel issues, gelatine peptides were found to modulate the abundance of gut bacteria such as *Akkermansia* and *Bifidobacterium*,[58] so it may be that gelatine peptides can modulate the gut microbiota composition. There is some evidence suggesting that collagen supplementation may help ease certain digestive symptoms, such as bloating, by supporting the integrity of the gut lining..[59] To help support and repair your gut lining, you may wish to try making your own broth (see page 37) and consuming it regularly. It is delicious as a warming drink or can be added to soups and stews. In this book, I have included many recipes that feature bone broth.

Protein is particularly important for the health of the gut lining. The amino acid glutamine is the preferred fuel for intestinal cells, and high-protein foods are a good source of glutamine. It can be found in a variety of foods, both animal and plant-based, including meat, fish, eggs, dairy products, cabbage, spinach, beets and certain wholegrains. Glutamine has been shown to help with leaky gut (see page 7) in several ways.[60] It promotes the proliferation of intestinal cells, regulates tight junction proteins (tight junctions are structures that seal the spaces between the cells lining the gut, allowing nutrients to pass in and out while preventing harmful substances from entering the bloodstream) and suppresses pro-inflammatory signalling pathways, which are crucial for maintaining the integrity of the gut barrier. If you wish, you can purchase glutatmine as a powdered supplement which can be added to drinks.

There are many other important nutrients for repairing the gut. They include vitamin D (mainly from sunlight, but also found in oily fish, liver, eggs, mushrooms), vitamin A (eggs, liver), beta-carotene (orange fruits and vegetables, dark green leafy vegetables) and zinc (meat, seafood, pumpkin seeds). To enhance the absorption of beta-carotene, add some fat to your meal; for example, include avocado or some oil in a dish containing carrots or kale.

Leaky gut is often associated with intestinal inflammation, oxidative stress (the production of free radicals) and the depletion of antioxidant reserves in the intestinal mucosa (which lines the small and large intestines). Including anti-inflammatory foods and those rich in antioxidants may be beneficial.

Quercetin[61] is a naturally occurring flavonoid with antioxidant and anti-inflammatory properties, and it also appears to support the gut barrier. Foods that are rich in quercetin include peppers, apples, onions, berries, capers and cacao powder.

N-acetyl-cysteine (NAC)[62] is an antioxidant and precursor for the production of glutathione, an essential antioxidant that can reduce oxidative damage and lower inflammation. NAC converts into cysteine, an amino acid found in protein foods such as poultry, fish and meat. Ensuring your diet is rich in quality proteins, therefore, helps with glutathione production.

Omega-3 fats play a key role in gut healing and can help to lower inflammation. In this book I have included a number of recipes that use omega-3-rich oily fish, and also some that use flaxseed and chia seeds, which are both sources of the parent omega-3 fatty acid known as alpha-linolenic acid.

In Step 3 Repopulate, I discussed the importance of beneficial bacteria. Probiotics can help modulate gut microbiota composition and improve gut barrier function, reducing inflammation. So, throughout Step 4 Repair continue to consume the fermented foods and prebiotic-rich foods described in Step 3. Other nutrients that can be helpful for lowering inflammation include turmeric and ginger.

If you have an irritated gut lining and experience heartburn or discomfort, you may wish to try making a drink or smoothie using soothing herbs such as aloe vera, slippery elm powder, marshmallow root or deglycerized liquorice. Try the Green Gut Healer recipe on page 59.

Consider supplements

There are a number of supplements that may be beneficial. In addition to glutamine, you could try taking colostrum (if you can tolerate dairy). Colostrum is milk produced by grass-fed cows shortly after birthing. It contains growth factors, a number of immunoglobulins, the immune modulating molecule lactoferrin and several vitamins and minerals, all of which may help lower inflammation and support the gut barrier.[63] Colostrum powder is readily available as a supplement and is a delicious addition to drinks and recipes. Collagen,[64] which is also available as a powder, is important for the health of the gut barrier, too.

Research has demonstrated that the SCFA butyrate significantly supports gut health. Butyrate[65] enhances the integrity of the gut barrier, reducing leaky gut. It is also protective and has anti-inflammatory effects on the intestinal mucosa.

Step 5: Rebalance

Our lifestyle habits have an enormous influence on our digestive system and health. During Step 5, we want to rebalance our body and mind, addressing stress management, exercise and sleep in particular. Maintain your digestive health during this stage by consuming sufficient fibre and probiotics, plus lots of anti-inflammatory fruit and vegetables. These are all included in various recipes in this book.

Managing stress

Most of us are well aware that our emotions can have a profound effect on our digestion. Stress, in particular, affects our gut health and function.

Cortisol and other stress hormones can influence digestive secretions and muscle contractions, cause shifts in our gut microbiota (leading to dysbiosis) and promote inflammation and leaky gut. Stress can affect digestive functions by altering appetite, slowing nutrient absorption and disrupting the production of mucus and stomach acid. This can lead to symptoms such as nausea, constipation, diarrhoea and abdominal pain. Stress can also impact sleep (see page 26), which can further affect our gut health.

As we know, our gut–brain axis (see page 8) is bidirectional, meaning imbalances in the gut can impact our mood and resilience to stress. Recent research[66] has shown that consuming probiotic supplements and fermented foods can help reduce stress and anxiety, further highlighting the critical relationship between beneficial bacteria and mental health.

For tackling stress, there are several adaptogenic herbs that can help the body to adapt or cope with stress. Maca and ashwagandha are two examples. They are readily available as powders that can be added to recipes. Try drinking green tea, too. Green tea contains the amino acid L-theanine, which increases the activity of gamma-aminobutyric acid (GABA), a neurotransmitter known for its anti-anxiety effects. Other calming teas include holy basil, peppermint, passionflower, hops and lemon balm.

Increasing your intake of magnesium-rich foods may also be helpful during the Rebalance stage. Magnesium can aid relaxation and sleep, but it is rapidly depleted during times of stress or heavy exercise. Magnesium-rich foods include dark leafy greens, nuts and seeds, fish, avocado, banana, cacao powder and dried fruit.

Many people find various mind–body therapies beneficial. Eye movement desensitization and reprocessing (EMDR), cognitive behavioural therapy or hypnotherapy may be useful for reducing anxiety and stress; however, simply taking time for proper relaxation – engaging in activities such as yoga, box breathing and meditation, practising mindfulness or writing a gratitude journal – can also be a great help.

Box breathing is a simple breathing technique that helps regulate the breath, balance oxygen and carbon dioxide levels in the blood, and activate the parasympathetic nervous system, which promotes relaxation and digestion. Sit in a comfortable position with your back straight and shoulders relaxed. Breathe in slowly and deeply through your nose for a count of four, filling your lungs completely. Hold your breath for a count of four. Exhale slowly for a count of four, emptying your lungs fully. Hold your breath again for a count of four before beginning the next inhale. Repeat for two to three minutes.

Regular exercise, when practised alongside diet and stress management, can noticeably improve digestive symptoms.[67] Activities such as yoga[68] have been shown to alleviate IBS symptoms in particular. In addition, physical activity has been proven to reduce levels of inflammatory markers in IBD and support the health of the gut barrier.[69] Exercise helps to improve your psychological health – reducing stress, anxiety and depression – but if you are struggling with digestive symptoms, you may not feel like exercising. It is worth making the effort if you can, because even walking, particularly after a meal, can be effective in alleviating symptoms such as bloating.[70] It may also improve bowel motility and ease constipation.[71] Remind yourself that making exercise an integral part of your daily routine will play a key role in improving your digestive symptoms.

Mindful eating is one of the most effective things you can do to rebalance your mind and body. Take time over your meals, chew your food properly and maintain consistent eating patterns. Avoid eating large meals late at night, which may cause digestive symptoms and interfere with sleep.

Importance of sleep

Research has shown a strong connection between how well you sleep and digestive symptoms. This relationship is complex and involves the gut–brain axis, circadian rhythms (our body's natural 24-hour cycles) and melatonin levels. Circadian rhythms help regulate many of our bodily functions, including digestion and the activity of gut bacteria. Melatonin is a hormone produced by the pineal gland in the brain, primarily known for its role in regulating sleep/wake cycles. Some research suggests that people with IBS may have lower levels of melatonin or disruptions in the circadian rhythm, which could contribute to sleep disturbances. Poor sleep, irregular sleep patterns, shift work or jet lag can lead to imbalances in the gut microbiota making symptoms worse.[72] Lack of sleep can also increase sensitivity to pain and alter gut motility. Some studies have looked at the use of melatonin[73] to improve sleep quality and reduce the severity of IBS symptoms. If your sleep is disrupted, consider whether you need to lower you stress levels, as cortisol interferes with the production of melatonin. Some people find that soaking in a bath of Epsom salts is beneficial. Simply put 2 cups of salts in a warm bath and soak for 20 minutes. Taking additional magnesium (magnesium glycinate or threonate) at night may also be helpful, as may drinking herbal teas such as chamomile or valerian, or a warm glass of Montmorency cherry juice in the evening.

Here are some more tips:

- Be consistent with your sleep routine: go to bed and wake up at the same time every day, including at the weekend.
- Allow time in the evening to unwind: practise relaxation exercises and breath work, switch off electronics, write in your journal or meditate.
- Avoid caffeine in the afternoon: the half-life of caffeine is 5 to 6 hours.
- Cut out alcohol because it reduces sleep quality and can cause you to wake through the night.
- Keep the bedroom cool, dark and quiet.
- Consider taking supplements such as magnesium glycinate or threonate, glycine, L-theanine and ashwagandha.

How to Follow the Programme

The recipes in this book are designed to improve ongoing digestive symptoms and facilitate gut health. They are all gluten-free for ease, as many people with digestive symptoms find wheat and/or gluten problematic. This does not mean you have to follow a gluten-free diet (unless you are coeliac). If you know you can tolerate wheat or gluten, there is no need to exclude them unnecessarily. There are also recipes suitable for those following a low FODMAP diet. The long-term aim is to avoid overly restricting your diet, so if you are following a low FODMAP diet, seek support from a dietitian or nutritionist to guide you through the reintroduction stages.

To support the 5R approach, all the recipes are labelled according to the stages they cover. Many are suitable for more than one stage or, in fact, all the stages. If you know your triggers and/or are already taking steps to support your gut health, you may be able to use any of the recipes in the book. Alternatively, you can follow the five steps described above and select your recipes accordingly. Remember to personalize the 5R approach to suit your symptoms.

I have already mentioned that rebalancing the body and addressing stress, sleep and exercise are crucial throughout the gut restoration programme, so make those changes from the start. In the same way, you may find that you can include fermented foods and a greater range of fibre-rich foods straight away – if you don't bloat up when you eat them. It is important to listen to your body to determine which foods, and how much, you can tolerate.

The length of time you spend on each stage is up to you. Step 1 Reduce/Remove typically lasts 4 weeks. This gives you enough time to see if removing common trigger foods will reduce your symptoms. If you have inflammation or leaky gut, it may take several weeks for noticeable improvement, in which case you would spend longer on Step 4 Repair. As you work through the steps, remember the goal is not only to reduce symptoms but also improve overall gut health. This means you want to be moving toward a diet that includes plenty of variety, particularly plant-based foods such as fruits, vegetables, nuts, seeds, legumes and wholegrains.

Key principles
Get the basics right

Studies have shown that simple dietary and behavioural changes can be very effective for people with digestive symptoms. One comparison study found that following a Mediterranean, low FODMAP or gluten-free diet resulted in similar improvements in symptoms. However, people preferred the Mediterranean diet because it was less restrictive.[74]

Eat sufficient protein: Ensure that you include protein in most meals: a palm-size portion (or two eggs) is sufficient for most people. Protein from meat, fish, poultry and eggs is generally well tolerated by the digestive tract and will help support satiety, energy and overall health. As a number of dairy foods contain lactose, some people may find these problematic. Others may have an allergy toward casein, a protein in many dairy products. If you are consuming dairy, you may wish to select low lactose options and spread out your intake across the day.

Be mindful that many plant-based proteins contain fibre, fructans and GOS (legumes, for example) that may contribute to symptoms such as bloating. For this reason, you may wish to avoid legumes initially and reintroduce them in small amounts as symptoms improve. Useful low FODMAP sources of plant proteins include tofu, pea protein, tempeh, natto and Quorn. Nut and seed butters are generally well tolerated, with the exception of cashew and pistachio nuts, which are high in fermentable fibres (GOS).

Include fats and oils: Fats are an important part of a healthy diet. Those that are rich in monounsaturated fats (such as olives, avocado and some nuts) and omega-3 fats (present in oily fish, seafood, walnuts, hemp, chia seeds and flaxseed) are especially beneficial because of their anti-inflammatory properties. Animal fats such as butter/ghee provide butyrate and vitamins A and D, which are important for gut health. Saturated fats such as coconut oil and monounsaturated fats like olive oil and cold pressed rapeseed oil are useful for cooking. More heat-sensitive fats, such as flaxseed, chia and hemp oils, are recommended for dressings. If you find excess fat aggravates your symptoms, opt initially for some of the lower fat recipes.

Ensure plenty of vegetables: Vegetables are an essential part of a gut healthy diet and should form at least half of your plate at each meal. They are packed with vitamins and minerals, anti-inflammatory antioxidants, enzymes and soluble fibre. Try and include a good amount of colour and variety.

Be mindful of fructose: Many people with digestive symptoms notice they feel worse when they eat foods with a high fructose content. These foods include honey, agave syrup, fruit juices, blackberries, apples, cherries, peaches, plums, canned fruits in apple/pear juice and dried fruits. Remember, when a food contains both fructose and glucose, the ratio between these two sugars affects how well our bodies can absorb the fructose. We absorb fructose most efficiently when there is an equal or greater amount of glucose present in the food. Certain foods, such as those listed above, typically contain more fructose than glucose, which can be problematic for some people.

When eating such foods, try and spread your intake across the day. Avoid fruit smoothies that contain both milk and high fructose fruits because they may exacerbate your symptoms. If you notice an issue with fructose, select fruits such as kiwi, banana, citrus fruits (satsumas, clementines, grapefruit and so on), cantaloupe melon, blueberries, raspberries, strawberries, pomegranate and Sharon fruit.

Watch fructans: We know that fibre is beneficial for gut health, but too much can be problematic if you have a sensitive gut. Many fibre-rich foods such as wheat- and rye-based products are also high in fructans, a type of FODMAP that often contributes to digestive symptoms. For this reason, it is best to avoid these products while you are following the programme. Certain vegetables like garlic and onions are high in fructans, and may contribute to symptoms. I have suggested alternative ingredients in many of the recipes (for example, spring onions tops are low FODMAP, or try garlic-infused oil) or you can omit them if you prefer. Legumes such as beans and pulses contain a range of fermentable fibres, including fructans, so these are best avoided initially. You may find red split lentils and canned legumes easier to tolerate.

Include fermented foods: Fermented foods are an essential part of the programme. They provide the body with an array of beneficial bacteria and yeasts. Various studies[75] have shown IBS symptoms to improve when probiotic-rich foods, such as kimchi, sauerkraut and yogurt, are consumed regularly. Fermented foods have been seen to increase microbiota diversity and decrease markers of inflammation.[76] The aim is, therefore, to include fermented foods on a daily basis. Either make them yourself or buy them. Many of the recipes in this book include fermented foods.

Stay hydrated: Water is essential for digesting and absorbing foods, transporting nutrients, keeping cells functioning properly and removing toxins via the liver and kidneys. Not drinking sufficient water can make you constipated and sluggish. Aim for 1.5–2 litres (2.6–3.5 pints) of fluid daily. This can include broths, soups, tea, coffee, herbal teas, and green juices or smoothies.

Avoid alcohol throughout the programme because it can adversely affect the gut. Limit shop-bought fruit juices, especially apple and pear, which are high in fructose. Shop-bought smoothies also tend to be high in fructose. Caffeine can be beneficial but also problematic. Remember, caffeine may be useful for alleviating constipation, but many people find it aggravates the gut. Find your tolerance level, but if in doubt reduce your intake to one coffee a day or avoid caffeine altogether until symptoms improve.

Watch your overall carbohydrate load: Carbohydrates are a great source of fibre, but they may be a double-edged sword. If you have a sensitive gut and experience frequent bloating, reducing your overall carbohydrate intake may help alleviate symptoms. It is all about finding your tolerance level, because your long-term goal is to enjoy a wide range of carbohydrates without adverse effects. There is a good selection of recipes in this book that focus on starchy and colourful vegetables and fruit, as well as nuts and seeds. Many of the recipes have the option to include a grain such as wholegrain rice, quinoa, buckwheat or oats, which are all great sources of fibre but low in fermentable fibres.

Limit sweeteners and sugars: If you are struggling with digestive symptoms, reducing your overall intake of sugars may be beneficial. One study found that people with IBS-D who followed a 4-week starch- and sucrose-reduced diet reported relief of symptoms and improvement in their quality of life after 2 weeks.[77] Reducing overall sugar and starches in the diet has also been shown to improve the gut microbiome in people with IBS.[78] It is worth noting that honey and agave syrup can be problematic due to their high fructose content. If fructose is a trigger for you, it is better to use small amounts of maple syrup or table sugar.

Reducing or removing artificial sweeteners (sucralose, aspartame, acesulfame K, and saccharin) has been seen to improve many IBS symptoms, including diarrhoea, post-prandial discomfort, constipation and burning. It seems that artificial sweeteners may cause changes in the gut microbiome, which, in turn, appear to affect gut function.

Increase polyphenols: Polyphenols are naturally occurring compounds found in a wide variety of plants known for their antioxidant and anti-inflammatory properties. They can also act as prebiotics, supporting beneficial microbes in the gut. Polyphenol-rich[79] foods like blueberries have been shown to improve general wellbeing, as well as abdominal symptoms and pain in people with IBS. Polyphenol supplementation has also been seen to increase levels of beneficial bacteria, such as *Lactobacillus* and *Bifidobacterium* species, and inhibit pathogenic *Clostridium* species. For this reason, try to increase the range of polyphenol-rich foods in your diet. These include strawberries, raspberries, blackberries, cranberries, walnuts, pecans, chestnuts, olives, pomegranate, grapes, tea (including green tea), coffee, chocolate, apples and cherries.

Include anti-inflammatory foods: There are a number of foods known for their anti-inflammatory properties. Try to include them throughout the programme. Examples include green tea extract (matcha green tea powder), herbs (basil, coriander/cilantro, mint, oregano, parsley, rosemary), mushrooms (including shiitake mushrooms), oily fish (anchovies, mackerel, prawns/shrimp, salmon, sardines, trout), omega-3-rich seeds (chia seeds, flaxseed, hemp seeds, pumpkin seeds), pineapple (for its bromelain), papaya (for its papain) and spices (ginger, turmeric). Foods rich in monounsaturated fats (avocado, olive oil, macadamia nuts), polyphenols (berries, olive oil, tea, walnuts), probiotics (fermented foods), quercetin (apples, capers, chillies, onions), resveratrol (berries, red grapes) and vitamin D (eggs, full-fat dairy products, liver, oily fish) also have anti-inflammatory properties.

Think balance and variety: At each meal, at least a quarter of your plate should contain high-quality protein. Roughly half your plate should contain vegetables, including dark green leafy vegetables and lots of colour and variety. On the remaining quarter, add some starchy vegetables or wholegrains such as quinoa, wholegrain rice, butternut squash, sweet potato, carrots or beetroot/beets. Always include healthy fats. These may occur naturally in meat, fish, avocado or olives, for example, or you may prefer to drizzle a dressing over your food or cook your food in fat.

Supporting supplements

While certain supplements may be beneficial during the various programme steps, they are optional and should be viewed as secondary to getting the right diet and lifestyle in place. It is recommended that you see a healthcare practitioner to find the most suitable supplements.

Note If you are taking any medications, it is important to consult your doctor before starting any supplements.

Steps 1 and 2: Reduce/Remove, Replace

Microbial infection: If you suspect you have a microbial infection, please seek professional advice. Common antimicrobial agents that can be taken with your meal include oregano oil, berberine, garlic, grapefruit seed extract, caprylic acid, plant tannins and *Saccharomyces boulardii*.

Flatulence/distension/abdominal pain: Enteric-coated peppermint oil capsules with each meal.

To improve digestive secretions: Digestive enzymes with each meal and/or betaine HCL (do not take if you have heartburn, reflux, gastritis, stomach ulcers). Drink lemon and water or take digestive bitters before each meal. Other options include bile-supporting supplements and lactase enzymes (to support lactose digestion). If you suspect histamine intolerance, consider DAO enzymes with your meals.

Constipation: Supplement with psyllium seed husk daily, taken with a glass of water, or 1 tablespoon flaxseeds or chia seeds with a glass of water. Build up gradually and ensure sufficient fluid intake. Butyrate supplements such as sodium butyrate may be helpful. Other options include magnesium (such as citrate or oxide) at bedtime up to bowel tolerance (when the stools become loose) and/or 1–2g vitamin C in divided doses (500mg) throughout the day to bowel tolerance. Probiotics such as *Bifidobacterium lactis* BB-12/ *Bifidobacterium lactis* HN019 or *Lactobacillus rhamnosus* GG may relieve constipation, especially when combined with fibre.

Diarrhoea: *Saccharomyces boulardii*, take 1–2 capsules twice daily. *Lactobacillus acidophilus* NCFM has been studied in relation to diarrhoea and IBS symptoms; take 1–2 times daily.

Step 3: Repopulate

Mixed strain probiotic: Trial a course of probiotics – one that includes a combination of *Lactobacillus* and *Bifidobacterium* species, with at least 10 billion live organisms in each daily dose. *Saccharomyces boulardii* (probiotic yeast), take 1–2 capsules daily.

Step 4: Repair

Consider some of the following:

    Glutamine powder 5–10g twice daily
    Fish oil (EPA plus DHA) 1g
    Turmeric 500mg–1g daily

    Colostrum 5–10g 1–2 times daily
    Collagen powder 1–2 tablespoons twice daily
    Sodium butyrate (500mg–1g butyric acid) 1–2 times daily

Step 5: Rebalance

Consider any of the following:

    Rhodiola rosea or ashwagandha supplements
    Maca powder 1–2 teaspoons daily (can add to yogurt or smoothies)
    Magnesium glycinate 200mg 1–2 times daily
    L-theanine 200–400mg daily

Post plan: Maintain a healthy gut microbiota

It takes time and patience to reduce symptoms and improve overall gut health. As we know, the 5R approach is designed to tackle underlying factors that may be contributing to your symptoms, and ultimately the aim is for you to enjoy a diverse diet without overly restricting particular food groups. To maintain a healthy gut microbiota, introduce foods or food groups one at a time and monitor any symptoms. Many people like to do this at the weekend in case they experience a flare-up. Remember, the issue may relate to quantity, so you may not need to exclude your trigger food, just reduce the amount eaten in any one meal. If you have an adverse reaction, remove the offending food and go back to the plan until symptoms resolve. Try the food again in a different amount. This will help you understand your tolerance levels and feel more in control of your diet.

Five Weeks using the 5R Approach

Week 1: Reduce/Remove

This week we are focusing on reducing symptoms and removing foods that many people find problematic. Look at your overall dietary patterns and lifestyle, which may be contributing to your symptoms. If you need to follow a low FODMAP diet, select the recipes that are labelled as suitable for low FODMAP.

BREAKFAST	LUNCH	DINNER	SNACK
Light Digestive Lemon Aid (p. 58), Seeded Paleo Bread (p. 66) or gluten-free bread with poached egg and Chipotle Avocado Cream Spread (p. 168)	Restorative Chicken Noodle Soup (p. 87) with Seeded Paleo Bread (p. 66), oat cakes or gluten-free bread plus a leafy green salad	Cod with Mediterranean Herb Dressing (p. 131) and steamed vegetables. New potatoes or sweet potato (optional)	Barbecue Kale Crisps (p. 169) 2 kiwi fruit
Pumpkin & Cinnamon Paleo Granola (p. 68) with milk alternative or lactose-free milk and berries	leftover Chicken Noodle Soup with Seeded Paleo Bread or gluten-free bread plus a leafy green salad	Southern-Spiced Pulled Pork with Sauerkraut (p. 121) or with steamed greens. Add extra vegetables or salad if you like	Chipotle Avocado Cream Spread (p. 168) with vegetable sticks 2 kiwi fruit
Spiced Omelette (p. 78) or Tofu Scramble (p. 83) 2 kiwi fruit	leftover Pulled Pork with Sauerkraut, plus a mixed salad	Vegan Mexican Taco Bowl (p. 136)	Fennel & Poppy-Seed Crispbreads (p. 164) Blueberries with soy, coconut or low lactose yogurt
Yogurt or dairy-free yogurt with berries topped with Pumpkin & Cinnamon Paleo Granola (p. 68)	Broccoli & Watercress Cleanse (p. 92) with Chia, Flaxseed & Tomato Crackers (p. 167) and smoked salmon Or Spiced Omelette (p. 78)	Roasted Whole Salmon with Sweet Soy & Star Anise (p. 129) with steamed vegetables. New potatoes or cooked rice (optional)	Antioxidant Blast (p. 61) Rice cakes with peanut butter or other nut butter
Fluffy Coconut Blinis with Spiced Fruit Compote (p. 72)	leftover Roasted Salmon with mixed salad	Spinach, Tomato & Red Pepper Almond-Crusted Quiche (p. 138) with mixed salad and steamed vegetables	2 kiwi fruit Oat cakes or rice cakes with nut butter
Overnight Oats with Kiwi & Pomegranate (p. 82)	leftover Quiche with a salad of bitter greens	Tamarind-Glazed Mackerel (p. 104) with a mixed salad. New potatoes or cooked rice (optional)	Granola Fruit Bowl (p. 145)
Caramel Apple Chia Pot (p. 71)	Spiced Roasted Beetroot & Apple Soup (p. 88) with Fennel & Poppy-Seed Crispbreads (p. 164) and feta cheese	Mandarin Salad of Duck with Green Beans (p. 120) and a mixed salad	2 kiwi fruit

Week 2: Replace

During this week we are including recipes to support digestive secretions and add fibre and prebiotics.

BREAKFAST	LUNCH	DINNER	SNACK
Blueberry Almond Bread (p. 65) spread with nut butter or butter	Asian Coconut Broth with Prawn Dumplings (p. 91) with Chia, Flaxseed & Tomato Crackers (p. 167) or gluten-free bread	Chicken & Artichoke Salad with Roasted Garlic & Herb Dressing (p. 93)	Cherry & Coconut Layered Parfait (p. 148) or berries or yogurt
Creamy Turmeric Kefir (p. 59), Poached Eggs with Wilted Kale, Tomato & Dukka (p. 81)	leftover Chicken Salad	Grilled Prawns with Turmeric Lemon Aioli (p. 107) with steamed vegetables and side salad	Tropical Fruit Platter with Sweet Ginger & Mint Dressing (p. 147) with vegan nut cream (p. 48) or yogurt/coconut yogurt/soy yogurt
Light Digestive Lemon Aid (p. 58), Seeded Paleo Bread (p. 66) with smoked salmon and/or feta cheese	Asian-Spiced Lettuce Wraps (p. 94) with mixed salad and pickles or sauerkraut (pp. 51–55)	(fasting evening, optional) Turkey Meatballs with Roasted Tomato Chipotle Sauce (p. 119), with gluten-free pasta, spaghetti or courgette noodles	Beetroot Cumin Crisps (p. 170) yogurt with melon or berries
Tofu Scramble (p. 83)	Spiced Omelette (p. 78) with gluten-free bread or Chia, Flaxseed & Tomato Crackers (p. 167) and side salad	Purple-Sprouting Broccoli & Beef Kelp Noodle Salad (p. 100)	Citrus Mojito Kombucha (p. 58) yogurt with kiwi fruit
Buttermilk Waffles with Berries (p. 74) with vegan nut cream (p. 48) or coconut yogurt (p. 47) and fruit	leftover Purple-Sprouting Broccoli Salad	Sicilian Tabbouleh with Cauliflower Rice (p. 109) with poached salmon	raw herb cashew cheese (p. 49) or feta cheese with vegetable sticks yogurt with blueberries
Overnight Oats with Kiwi & Pomegranate (p. 82)	Sicilian Tabbouleh with Cauliflower Rice (p. 109) and cooked chicken breast or a boiled egg	Cumin-Spiced Halibut with Kale Salad (p. 132) and new potatoes or baked sweet potato	pickles or sauerkraut (pp. 51–55) crackers of choice
Smoked Salmon with Sweet Potato Apple Rösti (p. 77)	Kale Salad (p. 132) with cooked prawns/shrimp, chicken or pan-fried tofu/tempeh	Tempeh & Mushroom Bolognese (p.140)	Apple & Plum Crisp (p. 152) with yogurt (p. 46)

Week 3: Repopulate

With your meals this week, aim to include at least 120ml/4fl oz/½ cup in volume of fermented foods daily, as well as prebiotic foods as below.

BREAKFAST	LUNCH	DINNER	SNACK
Pumpkin & Cinnamon Paleo Granola (p. 68) with coconut yogurt or yogurt (pp. 47, 46) and berries	Vegan Mexican Taco Bowl (p. 136)	Hot-Smoked Trout with Pistachio Pesto Noodles (p. 103) and side salad	Citrus Mojito Kombucha (p. 58) sauerkraut and crackers
Poached eggs with Sauerkraut (p. 52) and wilted spinach or Tofu Scramble (p. 83)	leftover Hot-Smoked Trout with Noodles and side salad	Korean Spiced Beef with Kimchi (p. 126) and cooked rice or rice noodles	Lemon Balm & Berry Ice (p. 144) yogurt and berries
Pumpkin & Cinnamon Paleo Granola (p. 68) with yogurt and berries	Chicken & Artichoke Salad with Roasted Garlic & Herb Dressing (p. 93), side of pickles or sauerkraut	Lime-Marinated Salmon Salad with Fennel & Mango (p. 101) and new potatoes	Antioxidant Blast (p. 61)
Overnight Oats with Kiwi & Pomegranate (p. 82)	Spiced Roasted Beetroot & Apple Soup (p. 88), topped with yogurt, with Chia, Flaxseed & Tomato Crackers (p. 163) and smoked salmon or feta	Tempeh & Mushroom Bolognese (p. 140)	yogurt (p. 46) and fruit
Caramel Apple Chia Pot (p. 71)	Tofu Scramble (p. 83) with gluten-free or Paleo bread and mixed salad	Cod with Mediterranean Herb Dressing (p. 131), new potatoes or sweet potato	yogurt (p. 46) or vegan nut cream (p. 48) with fruit
Creamy Turmeric Kefir (p. 59), Matcha Green Tea & Lemon Breakfast Muffins (p. 62)	Spiced Roasted Beetroot & Apple Soup (p. 88), Chia, Flaxseed & Tomato Crackers (p. 167) with nut butter or feta cheese	Tofu Rice Bowl with Miso-Lemon Dressing (p. 141)	Sauerkraut (p. 52) and crackers
Overnight Oats with Kiwi & Pomegranate (p. 82)	Tofu Rice Bowl with Miso-Lemon Dressing (p. 141)	Braised Chicken with Green Olives & Preserved Lemon (p. 115) with Sauerkraut (p. 52)	Lemon Balm & Berry Ice (p. 144)

Week 4: Repair

During the repair phase, you may wish to include bone broth as a drink or in dishes. Continue to consume fermented foods and prebiotics to support the gut microbiota.

BREAKFAST	LUNCH	DINNER	SNACK
Green Gut Healer (p. 59), poached eggs with wilted spinach or Tofu Scramble (p. 83)	Restorative Chicken Noodle Soup (p. 87) with Chia, Flaxseed & Tomato Crackers (p. 167) and side salad	Beef & Liver Burgers with Wasabi Mayo (p. 128) with mixed salad and pickles or sauerkraut	Fruity Gummy Sweets (p. 163)
Pan-fried Indian-Spiced Liver (p. 75) or Pumpkin & Cinnamon Paleo Granola (p. 68) with yogurt and fruit	Restorative Chicken Noodle Soup (p. 87) with Chia, Flaxseed & Tomato Crackers (p. 167) and side salad	Cumin-Spiced Halibut with Kale Salad (p. 132), baby new potatoes or cooked rice	Apple & Plum Crisp (p. 152)
Creamy Turmeric Kefir (p. 59)	Harissa Roasted Tofu Salad (p. 110) with Chia, Flaxseed & Tomato Crackers (p. 167)	leftover Kale Salad with poached salmon or pan-fried tempeh	Mint & Chocolate Ice (p. 144)
Overnight Oats with Kiwi & Pomegranate (p. 82)	Tofu Scramble (p. 83) with gluten-free or Paleo bread and mixed salad	Tempeh & Mushroom Bolognese (p. 140)	Green Gut Healer (p. 59)
Antioxidant Blast (p. 61), Spiced Omelette (p. 78)	leftover Tempeh & Mushroom Bolognese (p. 140) and salad	Pomegranate Lamb Tagine with Cauliflower Rice (p. 125) or wholegrain rice or quinoa	Fruity Gummy Sweets (p. 163), bone broth (p. 37)
Buttermilk Waffles with Berries (p. 74) with yogurt (p. 46)	Spiced Omelette (p. 78) and salad	leftover Pomegranate Lamb with Cauliflower Rice or wholegrain rice or quinoa	Green Gut Healer (p. 59)
Overnight Oats with Kiwi & Pomegranate (p. 82) and yogurt	Tofu Scramble (p. 83) with gluten-free or Paleo bread and mixed salad	Cod with Mediterranean Herb Dressing (p. 131), baked sweet potato and side salad	Matcha Superfood Bites (p. 161)

Week 5: Rebalance

Try to gradually increase the range of foods eaten. Some of the recipes include adaptogenic herbs and foods rich in nutrients to support adrenal health.

BREAKFAST	LUNCH	DINNER	SNACK
Granola Fruit Bowl (p. 145)	Chicken & Artichoke Salad with Roasted Garlic & Herb Dressing (p. 93)	Pan-Seared Venison with Blueberries & Broccoli Mash (p. 122) with salad	Chocolate Maca Cream (p. 61) with protein powder
Chocolate Maca Cream (p. 61) with protein powder	Lentil & Goat's Cheese Salad with Roasted Red Peppers (p. 111)	Vietnamese Prawn & Bacon Fried "Rice" (p. 135)	Matcha Superfood Bites (p. 161)
Spiced Omelette (p. 78)	Tamarind-Glazed Mackerel (p. 104) with mixed salad and sauerkraut (p. 52)	Raw Pad Thai with Courgette & Carrot Noodles (p. 108)	Matcha Superfood Bites (p. 161)
Smoked Salmon with Sweet Potato Apple Rösti (p. 77)	leftover Pad Thai	Tofu Rice Bowl with Miso-Lemon Dressing (p. 141)	Apple & Plum Crisp (p. 152)
Breakfast Seed Bars (p. 67)	Tofu Rice Bowl with Miso-Lemon Dressing (p. 141)	Broccoli Pizza (p. 97) with mixed salad	Apple & Plum Crisp (p. 152) with yogurt (p. 46)
Chocolate Maca Cream (p. 61) with protein powder	leftover Paleo Pizza with salad	Roasted Whole Salmon with Sweet Soy & Star Anise (p. 129) with steamed vegetables	Breakfast Seed Bars (p. 67)
Overnight Oats with Kiwi & Pomegranate (p. 82)	leftover Roasted Salmon with salad and pickles (pp. 51–55)	Braised Chicken with Green Olives & Preserved Lemon (p. 115)	yogurt and berries

Basic Recipes

The recipes in the section are for healing staple foods that are essential to include during your programme. They appear in most of the recipes in the book.

Stocks and fats for cooking or serving

One of the most effective ways to nourish and heal your gut is to consume homemade bone broths daily and include plenty of healing fats in your diet.

5-STEP					DIETARY						
REM	REPL	REPA	REB		D	F	G	GR	P	S	SC

NUTRITIONAL INFORMATION PER 100ML/3½FL OZ/GENEROUS ⅓ CUP   Kcals 4, Protein 0.1g, Carbs 0.8g of which sugars 0.7g, Fat 0g of which saturates 0g Fibre 0g

Bone Broth

Makes: 3 litres/105fl oz/12 cups

1kg/2lb 4oz beef bones, or marrow
   bones or 1 chicken carcass,
   sawed or bashed into pieces

1 whole head of garlic, peeled (optional)

2 carrots, chopped

1 onion, quartered

2 celery stalks, chopped

1 bay leaf

2 tbsp apple cider vinegar

1 strip of kombu seaweed (optional)

A bone broth made from meat or chicken is an important nutrient-rich food to include daily in any gut-healing programme. The bone broth can be used as a drink or to add to dishes such as soups, stews and casseroles. For optimal nourishment, select bones from quality, organic, grass-fed animals, such as beef, pork, lamb or chicken. Bone broth is rich in calcium, magnesium and phosphorus, and it contains amino acids such as glycine, proline and arginine. The gelatine in bone broth is useful for healing the gut lining and supporting the digestion.

1   Put all the ingredients in a large flameproof casserole or saucepan with a lid. Add 3–4 litres/105–140fl oz/12–16 cups water to cover generously, then bring to the boil over a high heat. Reduce the heat to very low so that the stock is barely simmering. Cook for at least 8 hours and up to 24 hours. Top up with water, if needed, during cooking.

2   Strain the stock through a sieve/fine-meshed strainer. Cool and store in the fridge for up to 3 days. Once completely cooled, skim off the fat that rises to the top. (You can store the fat and use it to cook with, if you like.) The stock can also be frozen in batches for up to 1 month.

NUTRITIONAL INFORMATION PER 15G/½OZ/1 TBSP   Kcals 135, Protein 0g, Carbs 0g of which sugars 0g, Fat 15g of which saturates 10g Fibre 0g

Ghee

Makes: 375g/13oz/1½ cups

450g/1lb/1¾ cups unsalted butter

The cooking fat, ghee, is made by melting unsalted butter and removing the milk solids, resulting in a pure fat with a high smoke point. Ghee is remarkably stable for cooking, even at higher temperatures. It is rich in butyric acid, also known as butyrate, a short-chain fatty acid (SCFA), which is used by the cells of the colon to protect the integrity of the gut wall and lower inflammation in the digestive tract. It is also rich in a range of nutrients, including omega-3 and -9 essential fatty acids.

Ghee contains vitamins A, D, E and K2. It does not contain lactose and so is tolerated by those with lactose intolerance.

1   Put the butter in a saucepan over a medium-low heat and leave it to melt, without stirring. After melting, the butter will separate into three layers: foam will appear on the top layer; the milk solids will migrate to the bottom of the pan; and clarified butter will float between the two.

2   Simmer the butter for 5 minutes, or until the middle layer becomes fragrant and more golden. The milk solids at the bottom will begin to brown. Using a spoon, skim off the top layer of foam into a bowl and discard. Turn off the heat and allow the liquid to settle for 1 minute.

3   Carefully pour the golden central layer through a sieve/fine-meshed strainer into a clean glass jar, leaving the milk solids in the pan. Discard the milk solids. Ghee can be stored at room temperature for 1 week or in the fridge for up to 1 month.

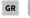
NUTRITIONAL INFORMATION PER 15G/½OZ/1 TBSP Kcals 113, **Protein** 0.3g, **Carbs** 0g of which sugars 0g, **Fat** 12.1g of which saturates 1.6g **Fibre** 0g

Mayonnaise

Makes: 300ml/10½fl oz/scant 1¼ cups

2 egg yolks at room temperature

a pinch of sea salt

½ tsp ground black pepper

150ml/5fl oz/scant ⅔ cup
   extra virgin olive oil

100ml/3½fl oz/generous
   ⅓ cup flaxseed oil

juice of ½ lemon

Egg yolks are nutritional powerhouses, rich in fat-soluble vitamins A, D, E and K as well as the protective antioxidants, carotenoids, lutein and zeaxanthin. Yolks also contain a range of minerals, including iron, zinc and B vitamins. By including a combination of olive oil and flaxseed oil you can optimize your intake of anti-inflammatory fats as well. Choose organic or free-range eggs.

Put the egg yolks, salt and pepper into a blender or food processor and process briefly to combine. With the machine running, gradually add the oils in a fine stream until the mixture is thick and emulsified. Add the lemon juice and pulse briefly to combine. Store in the fridge for up to 4 days.

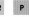
NUTRITIONAL INFORMATION PER 15ML/½FL OZ/1 TBSP Kcals 44, **Protein** 1.4g, **Carbs** 1.7g of which sugars 0.8g, **Fat** 3.5g of which saturates 0.7g **Fibre** 0.3g

Red Pepper & Chilli Vegan Mayonnaise

Makes: 275g/9¾oz/1¾ cups

130g/4½oz/1 cup cashew nuts

1 roasted red pepper/bell pepper

1 pickled red chilli, drained

½ tsp apple cider vinegar

2 tsp lemon juice

¼ tsp sea salt, or to taste

2 tsp tomato purée/paste

Rich and creamy, this is a delicious vegan mayo made with cashew nuts. Use it as a spread, a dip with crudités or for mixing into raw vegetables and salads.

If you have time, soak the nuts for 1–2 hours, then drain. Put all the ingredients into a blender or food processor and blend with just enough water to make it smooth and creamy. Season to taste. Store in the fridge for up to 4 days.

Nut and coconut milks

Milks made with coconut or nuts are a useful alternative to dairy. Many can be purchased ready-made, but it is also simple to make your own. Almond milk and coconut milk are particularly popular in recipes or as a dairy alternative in drinks. Almond milk is a good source of vitamin E and minerals, including zinc, which is beneficial for digestive function, and magnesium to aid relaxation. Coconut milk is a good source of medium-chain triglycerides (MCT) and contains lauric acid to support immune function.

Ideally, soak nuts overnight to make them more digestible. Always discard the soaking water. For a creamier milk, blend the nuts with less water. You can vary the flavourings and sweeten with a little stevia, dates or maple syrup, if you like.

5-STEP				DIETARY								
REM	REPL	REPA	REB	D	F	G	GR	P	S	SC	V	VE

NUTRITIONAL INFORMATION PER 100ML/3½FL OZ/GENEROUS 1/3 CUP   Kcals 89, Protein 3g, Carbs 1.6g of which sugars 1.3g, Fat 7.9g of which saturates 0.6g Fibre 0.2g

Almond Milk

Makes: 750ml/26fl oz/3 cups

125g/4½oz/heaped ¾ cup
   unblanched almonds

1 tsp vanilla extract (optional)

2–3 dried pitted dates, to taste
   (optional) (omit if low FODMAP
   – use stevia or maple syrup)

1   Soak the almonds in water for 8–12 hours, then drain. Put the almonds and vanilla in a blender or food processor and add 750ml/26fl oz/3 cups water. Add the dates, if you prefer a sweet milk. Blend until the mixture is smooth.

2   Line a colander or sieve/fine-meshed strainer with muslin/ cheesecloth, or use a nut bag, and put over a bowl or jug/pitcher. Pour in the liquid and allow it to drain into the bowl. Drink immediately or store in the fridge for up to 3 days. (The pulp can be dried and used in recipes: added to cracker or crispbread recipes instead of some of the seeds or nuts, or used to replace ground almonds in recipes.)

NUTRITIONAL INFORMATION PER 100ML/3½FL OZ/GENEROUS 1/3 CUP   Kcals 46, Protein 0.4g, Carbs 0.5g of which sugars 0.5g, Fat 4.7g of which saturates 4.1g Fibre 0g

Coconut Milk

Makes: 500ml/17fl oz/2 cups

70g/2½oz/1 cup coconut flakes

1 Put the coconut in a blender or food processor and add 500ml/ 17fl oz/2 cups boiling water. Blend for several minutes until the mixture is thick and creamy.

2 Line a colander or sieve/fine-meshed strainer with muslin/ cheesecloth, or use a nut bag, and put over a bowl or jug/pitcher. Pour in the liquid and allow it to drain into the bowl. Drink immediately or store in the fridge for up to 3 days. (The pulp can be dried and used in recipes: Paleo breads, muffins or granola.)

Fermented foods

If you look at any traditional culture, you will typically find fermented foods as part of their diet. Although fermentation was originally used as a means of preserving food, we now know that it also creates healthy, easily digested probiotic-rich foods.

Fermented foods provide beneficial bacteria, which support immune and digestive health. Organic fruit and vegetables, the soil and all plant matter are coated with the beneficial bacteria *lactobacillus* species and yeasts. When you ferment a food, you allow these bacteria to colonize and feed on the food.

This anaerobic process (or fermentation) does more than just preserve the food. It also makes the nutrients inside the food more bioavailable; for example, the amount of bioavailable vitamin C in sauerkraut is 20 times higher than in the same helping of fresh cabbage. This is because the vitamin C in fresh cabbage is bound in the cellulose structure of the plant, which can be more difficult to digest and absorb.

As communities of specific health-promoting bacteria grow, they consume sugars and produce valuable enzymes. Fermented foods are naturally rich in a wide range of beneficial probiotic bacteria and yeasts, making them an effective way to repopulate the gut.

Friendly bacteria are found in drinks such as kombucha, water kefir, milk or coconut kefir, yogurt and condiments such as sauerkraut and kimchi. For people avoiding dairy foods, kefir and a non-dairy yogurt can be made using nut milks and coconut milk; dairy milk is needed to feed the kefir grains every few days and can then be discarded. In the recipes in this book, coconut kefir is classed as vegan. If you are new to fermented foods, I recommend you start with just a spoonful to enable your digestive system to adjust. You can then gradually increase the amount you consume. Try to take 125ml/4fl oz/½ cup daily for optimal health. Use filtered water, if possible, in recipes for fermented foods.

Probiotic culture starters can be used to make fermented vegetable foods such as sauerkraut and kefir, and are a convenient way to boost the range of beneficial bacteria. These culture starters are easy to use at home and have been carefully developed to provide a safe range of beneficial bacteria.

NUTRITIONAL INFORMATION PER 100ML/3½FL OZ/GENEROUS ⅓ CUP   Kcals 13, **Protein** 0g, **Carbs** 3g of which sugars 1g, **Fat** 0g of which saturates 0g **Fibre** 0g

Kombucha

Makes: 750ml/26fl oz/3 cups

4–6 tea bags of green tea, to
  taste, or 1½ tbsp tea leaves

170g/6oz/¾ cup caster/granulated
  sugar, or coconut sugar

1 package of kombucha starter
  culture (SCOBY)

slices of orange or lemon,
  to serve (optional)

This refreshing fizzy drink is made from sweetened tea that has been fermented using a symbiotic colony of bacteria and yeast (known as SCOBY). It is rich in many of the enzymes your body produces for digestion and it aids cleansing and supports liver health. You can use any tea as the base of your kombucha, although green tea is particularly good. You can vary the flavourings – for example, by adding orange, lemon or lime to the brew. The starter SCOBY can be purchased online. The level of sugar and calories will vary depending on the length of time it has fermented – the SCOBY feeds on the sugar. Do not use metal equipment or utensils when making kombucha as this can affect the natural bacteria – use wooden or plastic spoons and plastic or glass bowls.

1   Put the tea bags in a 1 litre/35fl oz/4 cup sterilized glass jar and add the sugar. Pour over 750ml/26fl oz/3 cups boiling water. Stir well with a plastic spoon and allow the mixture to cool for 1 hour or until it reaches room temperature.

2   Add the SCOBY. Cover the container with a cloth or muslin/cheesecloth and leave in a warm place for 3–14 days to brew – the length of time will depend on the temperature of the room. The liquid will become a little cloudier when ready. After 3 days, taste the brew. If it tastes fruity and not like tea, it's ready; if not, leave it another day and try again. Strain the mixture, but leave a little of the tea in the container with the SCOBY so that you can make another batch of tea to repeat the process. You can keep the ready-made brew in the fridge for up to 4 days. Serve with a slice of orange, if you like.

Kefir

The ancient cultured food, kefir, is rich in amino acids, enzymes, calcium, magnesium, phosphorus and B vitamins. It also contains several strains of friendly bacteria and yeasts, which in combination can dramatically improve digestive function and immune health. Kefir is made using a mother culture, known as "kefir grains". The grains digest sugar in a fermentation process. There are two types of kefir – milk kefir and water kefir. To get the full benefit of this probiotic drink, ideally take it every day. Do not use metal equipment or utensils when making kefir as this can affect the natural bacteria – use wooden or plastic spoons and plastic or glass bowls.

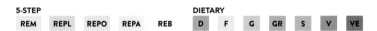

5-STEP REM REPL REPO REPA REB   **DIETARY** D F G GR S V VE

NUTRITIONAL INFORMATION PER 100ML/3½FL OZ/GENEROUS 1/3 CUP   Kcals 66, Protein 3.2g, Carbs 4.6g of which sugars 4.5g, Fat 3.9g of which saturates 2.4g Fibre 0g

Milk Kefir

Makes: 1 litre/35fl oz/4 cups

1 sachet of milk kefir grains

1 litre/35fl oz/4 cups organic full-fat milk or full-fat coconut milk

You can make kefir using organic dairy milk, or nut milks or coconut milk. If making coconut milk kefir, you will need to refresh the kefir grains in cow's milk after 4–5 batches to enable it to feed and grow. As the milk is fermented over 24 hours, it contains very little lactose and so may be tolerated by some people following a low FODMAP diet (see page 11).

1   Put the kefir into a 1 litre/35fl oz/4 cup sterilized glass jar and pour over the milk. Stir well using a wooden spoon. Cover with a lid or cloth and leave to ferment in a warm place, away from direct sunlight, for 24–30 hours. Do not seal the lid, as the gas can build up as it ferments. The milk will separate to form the kefir liquid at the bottom.

2   Strain through a plastic sieve/fine-meshed strainer into a clean jar and reserve the grains. After straining, put the grains straight back into a clean jar without washing them first. Add fresh milk to the grains to make the next batch. Store the prepared kefir in the fridge for up to 4 days.

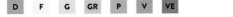
NUTRITIONAL INFORMATION PER 100ML/3½FL OZ/GENEROUS ⅓ CUP   Kcals 14, Protein 0g, Carbs 3.4g of which sugars 1.8g, Fat 0g of which saturates 0g Fibre 0g

Water Kefir

Makes: 750ml/26fl oz/3 cups

750ml/26fl oz/3 cups boiling water

70g/2½oz/scant ⅓ cup caster/
    granulated sugar

1 sachet of water kefir grains

juice of ½ lemon

1 thin slice of root ginger, peeled

You can introduce various beneficial herbs or flavours to water kefir to turn it into a variety of probiotic beverages; for example, try adding a herbal tea bag or some fresh berries to the kefir to add flavour.

1   Leave the water to cool until warm. Pour it into a 1 litre/35fl oz/ 4 cup sterilized glass jar. Add the sugar and stir to dissolve, using a wooden spoon. Add the water kefir grains, lemon and ginger, then stir.

2   Cover the jar and allow the water kefir to ferment at room temperature for 24–72 hours depending on the strength you prefer and the temperature of your home. Do not seal the lid as the gas can build up as it ferments.

3   Strain the water kefir grains, lemon and ginger through a nylon sieve/fine-meshed strainer over a clean jug/pitcher and bottle the liquid in smaller containers. Transfer the grains to a clean jar to start the process again. Allow the smaller bottles to rest for another 24–48 hours to continue fermentation and to produce natural carbonation.

Yogurt

Fermenting homemade yogurt for 24 hours reduces the lactose content of the milk and ensures that it is probiotic rich. Make sure you sterilize your yogurt containers. Homemade fermented yogurt is suitable for low FODMAP diets (see page 11); however, many commercial yogurts may be higher in lactose so watch your tolerance level if you are sensitive to lactose.

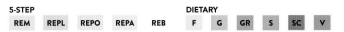

NUTRITIONAL INFORMATION PER 100G/3½OZ/HEAPED 1/3 CUP   Kcals 62, Protein 3.1g, Carbs 4.3g of which sugars 4.2g, Fat 3.6g of which saturates 2.3g Fibre 0g

Yogurt

Makes: about 990g/2lb 3oz/4 cups

1 litre/35fl oz/4 cups organic
   goat's or cow's milk

3 tbsp live plain yogurt or a
   commercial yogurt starter

1   Heat the milk in a saucepan over a medium-high heat to just below boiling point. Simmer for 2 minutes – do not boil. Remove from the heat and leave to cool down until the temperature is about 38–40°C/100–104°F. This should feel warm on the skin. Add the yogurt and stir well. Transfer to a yogurt maker or pour into a clean, dry vacuum flask. Leave the milk to ferment for 24 hours. After fermentation, stir well and put the yogurt in the fridge.

2   To thicken the yogurt, strain off some of the liquid. Put a piece of muslin/cheesecloth in a sieve/fine-meshed strainer set over a large bowl. Pour the yogurt into the lined sieve and leave it for several hours as the excess liquid drips through. The longer you leave it in the sieve, the thicker the yogurt will be. Store in the fridge for up to 5 days.

NUTRITIONAL INFORMATION PER 100G/3½OZ/HEAPED ⅓ CUP   Kcals 24, Protein 0.7g, Carbs 4.6g of which sugars 4.5g, Fat 0.3g of which saturates 0.2g Fibre 2g

Coconut Yogurt

Makes: about 800g/1lb 12oz/scant 3½ cups

2 × 400ml/14fl oz cans full-
   fat coconut milk

1 tbsp agar-agar flakes or gelatine

½ tsp probiotic powder, yogurt
   starter kit or 4 tbsp live yogurt

Use agar-agar flakes for a vegetarian version or gelatine to create a thick, creamy set yogurt.

1   Heat the coconut milk and agar-agar in a saucepan over a medium-high heat to just below boiling point. Simmer for 2 minutes and stir well to dissolve the agar-agar. Remove from the heat and leave to cool to room temperature. Stir in the probiotic powder.

2   Transfer to a yogurt maker or pour into a clean, dry vacuum flask. Leave the milk to ferment for 12–24 hours – the longer you leave it the more sour it will taste. After fermentation, stir well and put the yogurt in the fridge to firm up. Store in the fridge for up to 5 days.

NUTRITIONAL INFORMATION PER 100G/3½OZ/HEAPED ⅓ CUP   Kcals 141, Protein 4.7g, Carbs 5.6g of which sugars 2.1g, Fat 11.1g of which saturates 0.9g Fibre 2g

Almond Yogurt

Makes: 625g/1lb 6oz/2½ cups

125g/4½oz/heaped ¾ cup
   unblanched almonds

500ml/17fl oz/2 cups coconut
   water or water

1 tbsp maple syrup or honey

½ tsp probiotic powder, or yogurt
   starter kit or 3 tbsp plain yogurt

Use maple syrup to make this low FODMAP.

Soak the almonds for 12 hours, then drain. Put all the ingredients in a blender or food processor and blend until smooth and creamy. Pour into a 1 litre/35fl oz/4 cup sterilized glass jar, and leave on the worktop in a warm part of the room for 9–12 hours. It should now taste slightly sour. Store, covered, in the fridge for up to 1 week.

NUTRITIONAL INFORMATION PER 100ML/3½FL OZ/GENEROUS ⅓ CUP   Kcals 371, **Protein** 10.5g, **Carbs** 23.6g of which sugars 2.6g, **Fat** 28.5g of which saturates 5.6g **Fibre** 2g

Vegan Nut Cream

Makes: 125ml/4fl oz/½ cup

130g/4½oz/1 cup cashew nuts

1 tsp vanilla extract

1–2 tbsp sweetener, such as xylitol, maple syrup, honey or coconut syrup, to taste

2–4 tbsp water kefir or water

Any nut can be used to make this cream, but almonds and cashew nuts are particularly good. Use orange or lemon juice instead of water for a flavoured cream. For a savoury version, omit the vanilla and replace the sweetener with lemon juice, then season with salt and pepper – you can add a little tomato purée/paste, too, if you like. For a low FODMAP option, use almonds instead of cashews and maple syrup to sweeten.

Soak the cashew nuts in water for 2 hours, then drain. Put the nuts, vanilla and sweetener into a blender or food processor and add 2 tablespoons of the water kefir. Process until creamy. Add a little more liquid if needed to create a thick, creamy consistency. Store in the fridge for up to 4 days.

NUTRITIONAL INFORMATION PER 100G/3½OZ/¼ CUP   Kcals 279, Protein 10.7g, Carbs 9.6g of which sugars 2.1g, Fat 21.9g of which saturates 4.3g Fibre 2.3g

Raw Herb Cashew Cheese

Makes: 290g/10¼oz/2¼ cups

250g/9oz/scant 2 cups cashew nuts

120ml/4fl oz/½ cup water

½ tsp garlic salt

1 tbsp nutritional yeast flakes

zest of 1 lemon

1 tbsp lemon juice

2 probiotic capsules or ¼ tsp
    probiotic powder

2 tbsp finely chopped dill

2 tbsp finely chopped chives

finely chopped mixed herbs
    to serve (optional)

You can use this tasty fermented food as a snack or as a topping for a Paleo pizza or crackers.

1   Soak the cashew nuts in water for 4 hours, then drain. Put all the ingredients except the herbs into a blender or food processor and blend until smooth. Stir in the herbs.

2   Spoon the cheese into a 500ml/17fl oz/2 cup sterilized jar or container and ferment for 12–24 hours at room temperature, according to taste – the longer you leave it the slightly more sour it will taste. Serve as it is or shape it into a log and roll it in chopped herbs. Store in the fridge for up to 4 days.

Fermented pickles

Many shop-bought pickles use vinegar rather than the traditional method of salting, and because they are typically not fermented they do not provide probiotic bacteria, unlike home-fermented pickles. Probiotic cultures produced during lactic acid fermentation of vegetables are known to have many health benefits, including improving digestive health and immune health, lowering inflammation and protecting against microbial infections. Homemade pickled vegetables are also a good source of soluble fibre, making them ideal for bowel motility.

You can pickle most vegetables, and for additional benefits and flavour you can add spices, such as turmeric, and garlic or herbs. Use organic, fresh vegetables in season, if possible, when preparing pickles. Always wash and dry them thoroughly.

Homemade pickles are simply sliced or chopped vegetables, herbs and spices submerged in brine and tightly packed into a sterilized jar. The liquid must cover the vegetables. The lid is set loosely on top of the jar – don't seal it during fermentation.

To further boost the levels of beneficial bacteria, you can use a vegetable starter culture (available from online suppliers). Simply dissolve the starter in water, or according to the package instructions, and add to the prepared vegetable. Another alternative is to add 60ml/2fl oz/¼ cup whey to the vegetable and use it in the same way as the vegetable starter culture.

Leave the jar undisturbed at room temperature to ferment. You'll know that fermentation has begun when you see bubbles rising to the top of the jar and the water becomes cloudy. It generally takes between 3 and 10 days before the pickles are done. Taste the pickles during this time to see if they are ready. When making sauerkraut, fermentation may take up to 3 weeks. Taste regularly during fermentation from day 3.

Once fermented, store the pickles in the fridge for up to 1 month.

NUTRITIONAL INFORMATION PER 100G/3½OZ/²/₃ CUP Kcals 6, Protein 0.6g, Carbs 0.8g of which sugars 0.7g, Fat 0.2g of which saturates 0g Fibre 1.1g

Pickled Dill Cucumber

Makes: 1 × 1 litre/35fl oz/4 cup jar

2 cucumbers, sliced

2 garlic cloves, peeled

2 dill sprigs

1 tsp dill seeds

½ tsp black peppercorns

½ tsp coriander seeds

¼ tsp mustard seeds

a large pinch of dried chilli/
   hot pepper flakes

1 tbsp sea salt

a wedge of onion, if needed

These pickles make a tasty accompaniment to dishes and contain beneficial bacteria to support gut healing.

1   Pack the cucumber slices tightly into a 1 litre/35fl oz/4 cup sterilized sealable glass jar. Add the garlic, dill sprigs and seeds and the spices on top. Put 500ml/17fl oz/2 cups water in a jug/pitcher and stir in the salt. Stir until the salt has dissolved.

2   Pour this brine over the pickles, leaving about 2.5cm/1in of space between the brine and the top of the jar. All the cucumber must be fully submerged in the brine. If needed, put an onion wedge on the top of the cucumber to help to keep it submerged.

3   Cover the jar with the lid, but do not seal. Leave at room temperature for 3 days. Test a pickle on day 3. If it is to your liking, put the jar in the fridge to stop the fermentation process. If not, continue to ferment for a further day or two.

4   Seal and store in the fridge for up to 1 month.

NUTRITIONAL INFORMATION PER 100G/3½OZ/²/3 CUP   Kcals 29, Protein 1.5g, Carbs 5.1g of which sugars 4.9g, Fat 0.5g of which saturates 0.1g Fibre 2.7g

Sauerkraut

Makes: 1 × 1 litre/35fl oz/4 cup jar

1 cabbage, such as savoy or
  napa, finely shredded

3 carrots, grated or finely chopped

2 shallots, finely chopped

2 tbsp sea salt

1 handful of washed sea vegetables,
  such as dulse (optional)

2 garlic cloves, chopped

1 tsp caraway seeds

2 tsp fennel seeds

vegetable starter culture (optional)

Unlike many shop-bought versions, homemade sauerkraut is raw and therefore richer in beneficial enzymes and probiotic bacteria. You can vary the vegetables according to taste.

1   Put the cabbage, carrots and shallots in a large mixing bowl. Put 120ml/4fl oz/½ cup warm water in a small bowl and add the salt. Stir until the salt has dissolved.

2   Pour this brine over the vegetables and massage into the mixture using your hands. Leave at room temperature overnight to soften.

3   The following day, if using sea vegetables, soak them in water for 15 minutes, then drain and chop them. Leave to one side.

4   Drain the vegetables, reserving the brine. Stir the garlic and caraway and fennel seeds into the cabbage mixture and add the sea vegetables and vegetable starter, if using, or according to the package instructions. Mix well.

5   Tightly pack the mixture into a 1 litre/35fl oz/4 cup sterilized sealable glass jar. Pour over the reserved brine and press the mixture firmly so that there is no trapped air and the cabbage is covered in liquid. Cover the jar with the lid, but do not seal it. Leave the jar in a warm place for 3–4 days to ferment, then taste. If it is slightly vinegary, it is ready, otherwise leave it to continue fermenting, tasting it every few days. It can take up to 3 weeks to reach the correct level of fermentation, depending on the temperature of the room. Seal and store in the fridge for up to 1 month.

NUTRITIONAL INFORMATION PER 100G/3½OZ/²/₃ CUP   Kcals 27, Protein 1.2g, Carbs 5.2g of which sugars 5g, Fat 0.4g of which saturates 0g Fibre 2.5g

Red Cabbage & Beetroot Sauerkraut

Makes: 1 × 500ml/17fl oz/2 cup jar

½ red cabbage, finely shredded

1 beetroot/beet, grated

1 ripe pear, cored, peeled and chopped

1 tsp fennel seeds or caraway seeds

5cm/2in piece of root ginger,
   peeled and grated

1 tsp sea salt, plus extra if needed

vegetable starter culture (optional)

Beetroot is an ideal addition to support bile health, and this sauerkraut tastes deliciously sweet.

1   Put the vegetables, pear, seeds and ginger in a large bowl, add the salt and massage into the mixture using your hands for 2–3 minutes. Leave at room temperature, mixing occasionally for 1–2 hours, until the cabbage has wilted and released a little liquid.

2   Transfer the mixture to a 500ml/17fl oz/2 cup sterilized sealable glass jar. If using the starter culture, add to the mixture with 60ml/2fl oz/¼ cup water, or according to the package instructions. Press the mixture down firmly to pack it tightly. If the juices don't cover the mixture, add more salted water (using 1 teaspoon sea salt for each 250ml/9fl oz/1 cup water). Make sure the liquid covers the vegetables.

3   Cover the jar with the lid, but do not seal it. Leave the jar in a warm place for 3–4 days to ferment, then taste. If it is slightly sour, it is ready, otherwise leave it to continue fermenting, tasting it every few days. It can take up to 3 weeks to reach the correct level of fermentation, depending on the temperature of the room. Seal and store in the fridge for up to 1 month.

NUTRITIONAL INFORMATION PER 100G/3½OZ/²/₃ CUP   Kcals 26, Protein 0.7g, Carbs 5.6g of which sugars 5g, Fat 0.1g of which saturates 0g Fibre 1.9g

Speedy Kimchi

Makes: 1 × 500ml/17fl oz/2 cup jar

1 napa cabbage or Chinese cabbage,
    chopped into bite-size pieces

60g/2¼oz/¼ cup sea salt

1 tbsp dried chilli/hot pepper
    flakes, or to taste

vegetable starter culture (optional)

3–4 garlic cloves, to taste, crushed

2.5cm/1in piece of root ginger,
    peeled and grated

4 spring onions/scallions, sliced

2 tbsp fish sauce

½ onion

1 apple or pear, cored

1 tbsp coconut sugar or honey

Kimchi is a traditional Korean dish consisting of fermented chillies and vegetables, usually based on cabbage. It is a good accompaniment to meats and fish or to top salad. For a vegetarian option, omit the fish sauce.

1   Put the cabbage in a large bowl. Put 250ml/9fl oz/1 cup warm water in a small bowl and add the salt. Stir until the salt has dissolved.

2   Pour this brine over the cabbage, then give it a gentle toss, using your hands, to distribute the brine. Leave the salted cabbage to stand for 4 hours.

3   Drain the cabbage in a colander and rinse under cold running water to remove the excess salt, then transfer the cabbage to the rinsed-out bowl. Put the dried chilli/hot pepper flakes in a small bowl and add 2 tablespoons warm water and the vegetable starter, if using, or according to the package instructions. Stir gently with a spoon to create a paste, then stir this into the cabbage. Add the garlic, ginger, spring onions/scallions and fish sauce.

4   Put the onion into a blender or food processor and add the apple, sugar and 250ml/9fl oz/1 cup water. Blend until smooth, then add it to the cabbage.

5   Put on a pair of plastic gloves and massage the mixture using your hands to distribute the ingredients thoroughly. Transfer the cabbage and its liquid to a 500ml/17fl oz/2 cup sterilized sealable glass jar. Press the mixture down firmly to pack it tightly. Leave about 5cm/2in of space at the top of the jar. Cover the jar with the lid, but do not seal it. Leave the jar at room temperature for 24 hours. Seal and store in the fridge for up to 1 month.

NUTRITIONAL INFORMATION PER 100G/3½OZ/²/₃ CUP Kcals 5, Protein 0.2g, Carbs 0.8g of which sugars 0.8g, Fat 0g of which saturates 0g Fibre 1.7g

Turmeric-Infused Daikon, Red Radish & Ginger Pickle

Makes: 1 × 1 litre/35fl oz/4 cup jar

400g/14oz daikon radish, peeled

8 red radishes, thinly sliced

2.5cm/1in piece of root ginger, peeled
    and cut into very thin matchsticks

1 tbsp sea salt

1 tsp ground turmeric

1 Cut the daikon in half lengthways, then cut crossways into thin slices, using a mandoline if you have one. Pack the two types of radish into a 1 litre/35fl oz/4 cup sterilized sealable glass jar in alternate layers with the ginger.

2 Put 1 litre/35fl oz/4 cups water in a jug/pitcher and stir in the salt and turmeric. Stir until the salt has dissolved. Pour this brine over the vegetables, leaving about 2.5cm/1in of space between the water and the top of the jar. All the vegetables must be fully submerged in the brine. Cover the jar with the lid, but do not seal it. Leave at room temperature for 1–2 weeks or until it tastes slightly sour. Seal and store in the fridge for up to 1 month.

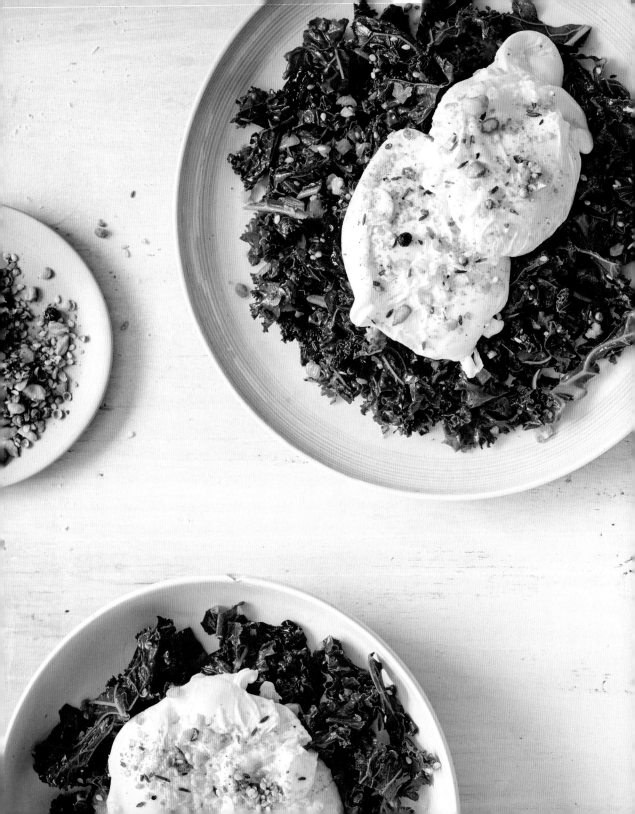

Juices, Smoothies & Breakfasts

Kick-start your day with a nourishing breakfast. The recipes in this chapter are rich in protein and healthy fats to stabilize blood sugar and energy levels. They also contain cleansing ingredients, nutrients and probiotics to soothe the digestive tract and calm inflammation. Try my Pumpkin & Cinnamon Paleo Granola, Caramel Apple Chia Pots or Buttermilk Waffles with Berries – or for a savoury option, make up a Spiced Omelette or Pan-Fried Indian-Spiced Liver. I have also included some grab-and-go dishes – Breakfast Seed Bars and Matcha Green Tea & Lemon Breakfast Muffins.

5-STEP

| REM | REPL | REPO | REPA | REB |

DIETARY

| D | G | GR | P | S | SC | V | VE |

NUTRITIONAL INFORMATION PER SERVING   Kcals 61, **Protein** 2.5g, **Carbs** 11.3g of which sugars 11.3g, **Fat** 0.5g of which saturates 0g **Fibre** 0g

Light Digestive Lemon Aid

Serves: 1

½ small fennel bulb

1 apple

1 lemon, peeled

1 handful of coriander/cilantro leaves

leaves from 4 mint sprigs

1 handful of spinach

1 cucumber

½ tsp probiotic powder (optional)

Put all the ingredients, except the probiotic powder, if using, through an electric juicer. Stir in the probiotic powder and serve immediately.

Gut Benefits

Coriander/cilantro has cleansing and detoxification properties. Fennel contains anethole, a volatile oil that stimulates the secretion of the digestive and gastric juices and reduces inflammation.

5-STEP

| REM | REPL | REPO | REPA | REB |

DIETARY

| D | G | GR | P | V | VE |

NUTRITIONAL INFORMATION PER SERVING   Kcals 47, **Protein** 0.4g, **Carbs** 10.6g of which sugars 3g, **Fat** 0g of which saturates 0g **Fibre** 0g

Citrus Mojito Kombucha

Serves: 1

leaves from 4 mint sprigs

3 tbsp lemon juice

2 tbsp orange juice

zest of 1 lemon

1 tsp vanilla extract

250ml/9fl oz/1 cup kombucha (page 43)

a few drops of stevia (optional)

1 handful of crushed ice

Bash the mint with the end of a rolling pin to release the flavour, then put it into a jug/pitcher and add the lemon and orange juices and the lemon zest. Add the vanilla and kombucha and stir to mix. Sweeten to taste, if needed, then pour into a glass and top up with ice. Stir and serve immediately.

Gut Benefits

Citrus aids the secretion of digestive juices and is a good source of vitamin C to support immune and adrenal function. Kombucha provides beneficial bacteria to support gut health.

NUTRITIONAL INFORMATION PER SERVING   Kcals 305, **Protein** 35.6g, **Carbs** 40.9g of which sugars 17.5g, **Fat** 3.3g of which saturates 0g **Fibre** 4.5g

Green Gut Healer

Serves: 1

½ banana

250ml/9fl oz/1 cup coconut water

¼ tsp probiotic powder

1 tbsp L-glutamine powder

1 tsp slippery elm powder

1 large handful of kale

½ ripe pear, cored and chopped

1 kiwi fruit, peeled and chopped

30g/1oz/scant ¼ cup vanilla vegan
   or whey protein powder

Put the banana into a blender or food processor and add the remaining ingredients. Blend until smooth and creamy. Serve immediately.

Gut Benefits

Glutamine is an essential amino acid that is known for its anti-inflammatory properties and is necessary for the growth and repair of the intestinal lining.

NUTRITIONAL INFORMATION PER SERVING   Kcals 146, **Protein** 1.6g, **Carbs** 27.8g of which sugars 26.4g, **Fat** 4.2g of which saturates 3.2g **Fibre** 4.5g

Creamy Turmeric Kefir

Serves: 1

5mm/¼in piece of turmeric root, peeled
   and grated, or ¼ tsp ground turmeric

150g/5½oz pineapple with core

1 tsp coconut oil

1 tsp shelled hemp seeds

1 tbsp lemon juice

250ml/9fl oz/1 cup coconut kefir
   or milk kefir (page 44)

Put all the ingredients into a blender or food processor and blend until smooth and creamy. Serve immediately.

Gut Benefits

Turmeric is one of the most potent natural anti-inflammatory spices available. Pineapple contains bromelain – which is particularly concentrated in the core – to support digestion and lower inflammation. Using kefir is a great way to inoculate the gut with beneficial bacteria.

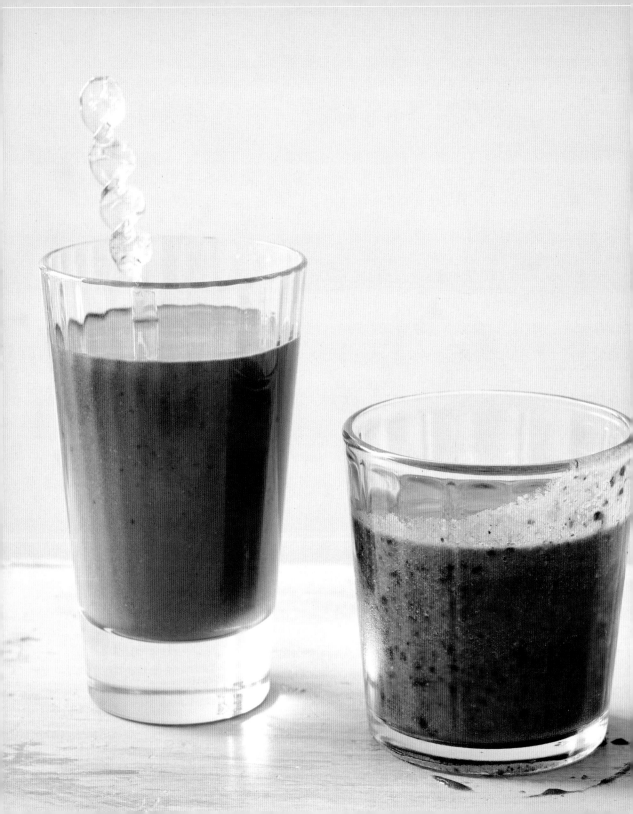

NUTRITIONAL INFORMATION PER SERVING   Kcals 261, **Protein** 6.8g, **Carbs** 27.5g of which sugars 1.3g, **Fat** 14.2g of which saturates 4.9g **Fibre** 3.5g

Chocolate Maca Cream

Serves: 1

1 tbsp cashew nut butter

1 tbsp raw cacao powder

1 large handful of mixed berries

1 tsp maca powder

1 tsp honey or maple syrup (optional)

30g/1oz/scant ¼ cup vegan or whey
   protein powder (optional)

250ml/9fl oz/1 cup almond milk
   or other milk alternative

Put all the ingredients into a blender or food processor and blend until smooth and creamy. Serve immediately.

Gut Benefits

Maca is a well-known adaptogenic herb (see page 25). The addition of protein helps to balance blood sugar levels, preventing energy dips and cravings, and it is also essential for repairing and healing the gut lining.

NUTRITIONAL INFORMATION PER SERVING   Kcals 115, **Protein** 5.3g, **Carbs** 13.6g of which sugars 2.6g, **Fat** 4.9g of which saturates 2.8g **Fibre** 4g

Antioxidant Blast

Serves: 1

1 tsp chia seeds

250ml/9fl oz/1 cup coconut water,
   or coconut kefir (page 44)

¼ tsp matcha green tea powder

2 handfuls of mixed berries

1 tbsp collagen powder (optional)

30g/1oz/scant ¼ cup vanilla vegan or
   whey protein powder (optional)

Put all the ingredients into a blender or food processor and blend until smooth and creamy. Serve immediately.

Gut Benefits

Chia seeds provide soluble fibre to improve bowel motility, and the addition of collagen provides easy-to-digest protein to nourish the gut.

NUTRITIONAL INFORMATION PER MUFFIN   Kcals 263, **Protein** 11.2g, **Carbs** 12.8g of which sugars 1.6g, **Fat** 20.1g of which saturates 4.4g **Fibre** 6.2g

Matcha Green Tea & Lemon Breakfast Muffins

Makes: 8 muffins

Preparation time: 15 minutes

Cooking time: 30 minutes, plus cooling

200g/7oz/1⅓ cups unblanched almonds

30g/1oz/¼ cup coconut flour

¼ tsp sea salt

½ tsp bicarbonate of soda/baking soda

1 tsp gluten-free baking powder

60g/2¼oz/⅓ cup xylitol, caster
    sugar or coconut sugar

zest and juice of 2 lemons
    (120ml/4fl oz/½ cup)

1 tbsp matcha green tea powder

60ml/2fl oz/¼ cup coconut milk or
    almond milk (pages 41, 40)

4 eggs, beaten

2 tbsp coconut oil, melted

1 tsp vanilla extract

1 heaped tbsp chia seeds

flaked/sliced almonds, to sprinkle

The ever-popular breakfast muffin is made grain-free and flavoured with lemon and matcha green tea powder to cram in plenty of anti-inflammatory antioxidants. They make a healthy breakfast or a snack on the go.

1   Preheat the oven to 180°C/350°F/Gas 4. Line an 8-cup muffin pan with paper muffin cases. Put the almonds in a high-speed blender or food processor and process until very fine. Add the coconut flour, salt, bicarbonate of soda/baking soda, baking powder, xylitol, lemon zest and matcha, then process to combine thoroughly. (Alternatively, tip into a large bowl and stir in the ingredients as above.)

2   Pour the lemon juice into a jug/pitcher and add enough coconut milk to make 170ml/5½fl oz/⅔ cup. Pour into the food processor or bowl followed by the remaining ingredients, except the chia seeds. Process, or stir, until smooth. Leave the mixture to stand for 5 minutes, then add the chia seeds and pulse, or stir, to combine.

3   Spoon the batter into the muffin cups and top each muffin with a few flaked/sliced almonds. Bake for 25–30 minutes until golden, cooked through and firm to the touch. Leave to cool for 5 minutes, then turn out on to a wire rack to cool completely.

Gut Benefits

Matcha green tea is packed with flavonoids – potent antioxidants known for their protective and anti-inflammatory benefits. It also contains the amino acid L-theanine, which has been shown to relieve anxiety and help the body cope with daily stress.

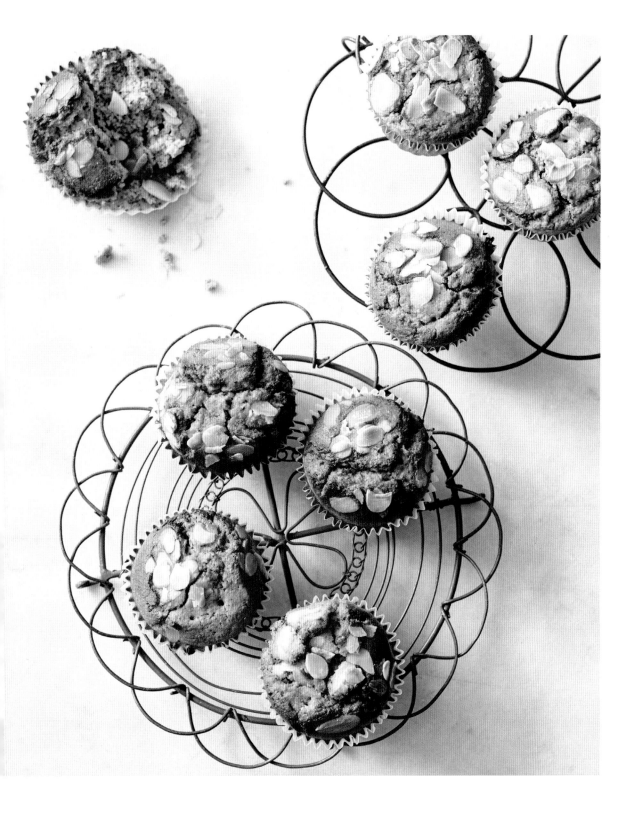

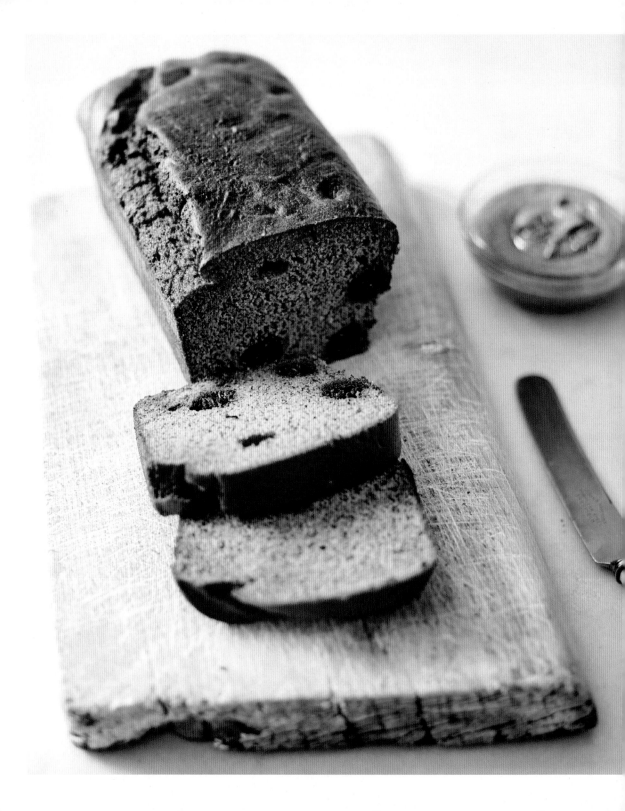

NUTRITIONAL INFORMATION PER SLICE   Kcals 256, Protein 6.2g, Carbs 14.6g of which sugars 6.8g, Fat 19.6g of which saturates 11.5g Fibre 4.8g

Blueberry Almond Bread

Makes: 1 × 900g/2lb loaf, 10 slices

Preparation time: 15 minutes

Cooking time: 45 minutes, plus cooling

100g/3½oz/½ cup coconut oil,
    plus extra for greasing

4 small ripe bananas, roughly chopped

4 eggs

130g/4½oz/½ cup almond nut butter

60g/2¼oz/½ cup coconut flour

1 tsp bicarbonate of soda/baking soda

2 tsp gluten-free baking powder

1 tbsp vanilla extract

1 tsp ground cinnamon

60g/2¼oz/⅓ cup frozen blueberries

Grain-free and wonderfully moist, this flavourful fruity bread is made with coconut flour. It is rich in fibre to support bowel health and stabilize blood sugar levels. The addition of nut butter gives it a further protein boost and a wonderful creamy texture.

1   Heat the oven to 180°C/350°F/Gas 4. Grease a 900g/2lb loaf pan and line it with baking parchment. Put the bananas into a blender or food processor and add the eggs, coconut oil and nut butter. Blend together.

2   Add the coconut flour, bicarbonate of soda/baking soda, baking powder, vanilla and cinnamon to the food processor or bowl. Blend, or mix together using a electric hand whisk/beater, then stir in the blueberries.

3   Spoon the batter into the prepared pan. Bake for 45 minutes or until golden and cooked through, and a skewer inserted into the middle comes out clean. Leave to cool in the pan for 5 minutes, then turn out on to a wire rack to cool completely. Slice to serve. Store in the fridge for up to 5 days or slice and open freeze until firm, then pack into freezer bags and freeze for up to 1 month.

Gut Benefits

As well as the nutrients and bowel-friendly fibre, this fruity bread also includes blueberries, which contain protective antioxidants. The nut butter is a good source of zinc and other nutrients that are beneficial for gut health.

NUTRITIONAL INFORMATION PER SLICE   Kcals 326, Protein 8.9g, Carbs 9.2g of which sugars 1.7g, Fat 28.2g of which saturates 10g Fibre 4.7g

Seeded Paleo Bread

Makes: 1 × 900g/2lb loaf, 10 slices

Preparation time: 15 minutes

Cooking time: 30 minutes, plus cooling

90g/3¼oz/scant ½ cup coconut
   oil, butter or ghee (page 38),
   melted, plus extra for greasing

250g/9oz/1²/₃ cups unblanched almonds

2 tbsp ground flaxseed

½ tsp salt

1 tsp bicarbonate of soda/baking soda

70g/2½oz/½ cup arrowroot

4 eggs, beaten

1 tsp lemon juice

120ml/4fl oz/½ cup coconut kefir
   (page 44) or coconut cream

2 tbsp mixed seeds, plus extra to sprinkle

Ground almonds make a nutritious base for this easy, grain-free bread. Use this to replace regular breads – it is ideal as a sandwich loaf or you can serve it toasted with Chipotle Avocado Cream Spread (picture on page 166) or poached eggs.

1   Preheat the oven to 180°C/350°F/Gas 4. Grease a 900g/2lb loaf pan and line the base with baking parchment. Put the almonds into a high-speed blender or food processor and process until very fine. Add the flaxseed, salt, bicarbonate of soda/baking soda and arrowroot, then pulse briefly to combine. (Alternatively, mix in a large bowl.)

2   Pour the coconut oil into the almond mixture and add the eggs, lemon juice and coconut kefir. Pulse, or stir, to mix well.

3   Stir in the seeds, then spoon the batter into the prepared pan. Sprinkle the top with the extra seeds. Bake for 25–30 minutes until golden and a skewer inserted into the middle comes out clean. Leave to cool in the pan for 5 minutes, then turn out on to a wire rack to cool completely. Serve in slices.

Gut Benefits

This easy-to-digest bread is fibre and protein rich as well as naturally gluten-free. If you can tolerate dairy, use butter or ghee, which is a useful source of butyric acid, known for its anti-inflammatory properties.

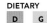 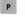
NUTRITIONAL INFORMATION PER BAR   Kcals 248, Protein 4.3g, Carbs 10.4g of which sugars 7.7g, Fat 20.9g of which saturates 7.8g Fibre 3.1g

Breakfast Seed Bars

Makes: 12 bars

Preparation time: 15 minutes

Cooking time: 30 minutes, plus cooling

70g/2½oz/⅓ cup coconut oil,
    plus extra for greasing

100g/3½oz/⅔ cup unblanched almonds

100g/3½oz/1 cup pecan nuts

2 tbsp desiccated/dried shredded coconut

1 tbsp lucuma powder

½ tsp bicarbonate of soda/baking soda

1 tsp maca powder (optional)

1 tsp ground cinnamon

100g/3½oz/½ cup pitted soft
    dried dates, chopped

2 tbsp coconut syrup or honey

70g/2½oz/heaped ½ cup mixed seeds
    (pumpkin, sesame, sunflower)

Many breakfast cereal bars are full of syrups and processed fats, but these grain-free seed bars are nutritious. They are ideal for a speedy breakfast when you're on the move or a healthy pre- or post-exercise treat. Freeze them and grab one as you go out.

1   Preheat the oven to 180°C/350°F/Gas 4. Grease and line a shallow 30 × 23cm/12 × 9in traybake pan with baking parchment. Put the almonds into a high-speed blender or food processor and add the pecans, coconut, lucuma, bicarbonate of soda/baking soda, maca, if using, cinnamon and dates. Process to chop the nuts and dates finely.

2   Put the coconut syrup and oil in a saucepan over a medium heat and warm through until the oil has melted. Add to the blender or food processor and briefly process to combine. Add the seeds and pulse into the mixture.

3   Spoon the mixture into the prepared pan, press down and smooth the top. Bake for 25–30 minutes until golden. Leave to cool in the pan, then turn out onto a board and cut into 12 bars. Store in an airtight container for up to 1 week or freeze for up to 1 month.

Gut Benefits

Adding seeds to these bars provides anti-inflammatory essential fats and zinc for helping digestive function. Coconut oil is rich in the antimicrobial and immune-supporting nutrients lauric acid and caprylic acid.

NUTRITIONAL INFORMATION PER 50G/1¾OZ/SCANT ½ CUP   Kcals 263, Protein 6.2g, Carbs 4.3g of which sugars 2.4g, Fat 24.5g of which saturates 6.6g Fibre 4g

Pumpkin & Cinnamon Paleo Granola

Makes: 820g/1lb 13oz/7 cups

Preparation time: 10 minutes

Cooking time: 30 minutes, plus cooling

70g/2½oz/1 cup coconut flakes

120g/4¼oz/scant 1¼ cups ground almonds

100g/3½oz/1 cup flaked/sliced almonds

60g/2¼oz/⅔ cup walnuts, chopped

120g/4¼oz/1 cup pumpkin
   seeds or mixed seeds

2 tbsp ground flaxseed

130g/4½oz /1¼ cups pecan nuts, chopped

120g/4¼oz/½ cup canned pumpkin
   purée or steamed and puréed
   squash or pumpkin

60g/2¼oz/heaped ¼ cup
   coconut oil, melted

2 tbsp maple syrup, coconut
   syrup or honey

2 tsp ground cinnamon

a pinch of sea salt

1 tbsp vanilla extract

Coconut and nuts form the base of this tasty grain-free granola with puréed pumpkin. If you use canned pumpkin, check that it doesn't contain sweeteners or sugars. If you like, add a spoonful of cocoa or cacao powder for a chocolate version or a spoonful of maca powder to support adrenal health. To make this suitable for a low FODMAP diet, use maple syrup. Serve with coconut yogurt, or plain thick yogurt, and fresh berries.

1   Preheat the oven to 180°C/350°F/Gas 4 and line a baking sheet with baking parchment. Put the coconut flakes in a large bowl and add the almonds, walnuts, pumpkin seeds, flaxseed and pecans. Mix well.

2   Put the pumpkin into a blender or food processor and add the coconut oil, maple syrup, cinnamon, salt and vanilla. Blend well to combine.

3   Pour the pumpkin mixture over the nut mixture and stir, using a wooden spoon, until thoroughly coated.

4   Spread the granola in a thin layer on the prepared baking sheet. Bake for 30 minutes or until lightly golden, stirring occasionally to prevent burning. Leave to cool. Store in an airtight container for up to 2 weeks.

Gut Benefits

The combination of coconut, nuts and seeds in this granola makes it nutrient rich with plenty of zinc, which the body needs for digestive function and healing. It's a good source of anti-inflammatory fats, too.

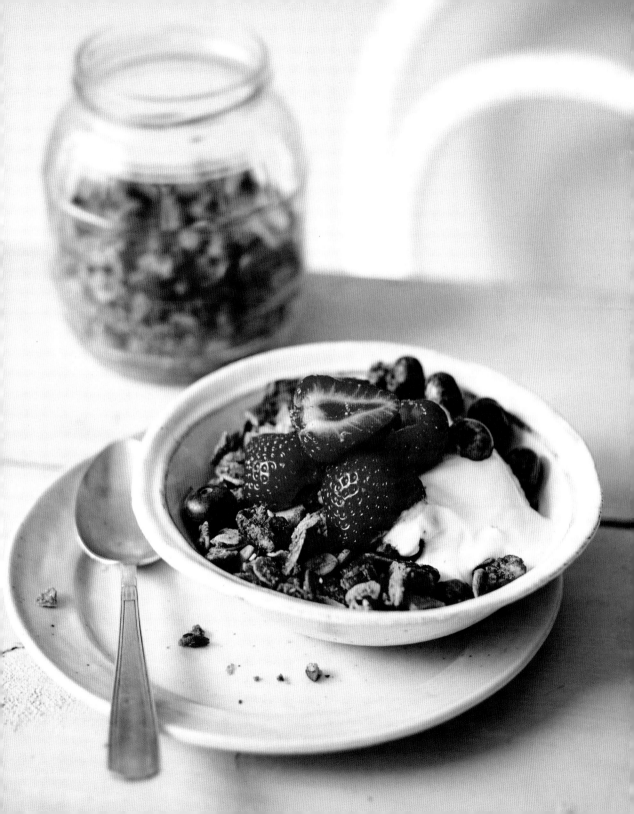

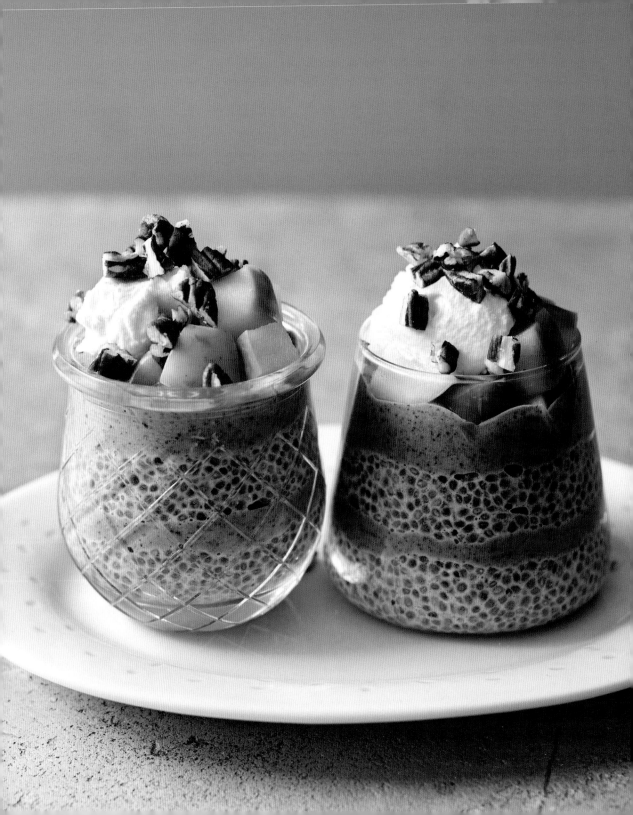

NUTRITIONAL INFORMATION PER SERVING   Kcals 493, Protein 11.6g, **Carbs** 61.7g of which sugars 23g, **Fat** 23.7g of which saturates 3.4g Fibre 16g

Caramel Apple Chia Pots

Serves: 2

Preparation time: 15 minutes, plus
   overnight soaking and 10 minutes
   standing

Cooking time: 5 minutes

300ml/10½fl oz/scant 1¼ cups
   almond milk (page 40)

½ tsp ground cinnamon

4 tbsp chia seeds

2 eating apples, cored and diced

coconut yogurt or yogurt (pages 47, 46)
   and chopped pecan nuts, to serve

CARAMEL

6 small pitted dates

2 tbsp lucuma powder, sifted (optional)

3 tbsp almond nut butter

1 tsp vanilla extract

100ml/3½fl oz/generous ⅓ cup almond
   milk or coconut milk (pages 40, 41)

Try this wonderful prepare-ahead sweet breakfast option that is equally delicious as a dessert or a filling snack. The chia and caramel can be prepared the night before and assembled in the morning. Lucuma, which is optional in the dish, is a maple-syrup-flavoured powder that adds a natural sweetness to dishes and is fibre rich. Maca powder would be a nice alternative or simply omit for a simpler version.

1   Put the almond milk into a blender or food processor and add the cinnamon. Blend to combine. Pour into a jug/pitcher and add the chia seeds. Stir well, then leave to soak in the fridge overnight.

2   To make the caramel, soak the dates in cold water for 10 minutes, then drain in a colander. Put all the ingredients into a blender or food processor and blend until smooth and creamy. Chill until ready to serve.

3   Put the apples in a small saucepan over a medium heat and add 100ml/3½fl oz/generous ⅓ cup water. Bring to the boil, then reduce the heat and simmer for 2–3 minutes until the apple is soft but still retaining its shape. Stir half the apple mixture into the chia seeds and almond milk.

4   Layer the chia seed mixture and the caramel between two glasses. Top with a spoonful of caramel and the remaining apple mixture. Top with a little coconut yogurt and chopped pecans, and serve immediately.

Gut Benefits

Stewed apple is renowned for its gut-healing properties. It is packed with polyphenols to support the growth of beneficial bacteria and pectin, a type of soluble fibre to aid bowel regularity. Soluble fibre is also present in abundance in chia seeds, making them ideal for tackling constipation.

NUTRITIONAL INFORMATION PER BLINI WITH COMPOTE   Kcals 104, **Protein** 4.5g, **Carbs** 9.4g of which sugars 4.3g, **Fat** 5.2g of which saturates 2.8g **Fibre** 3.8g

Fluffy Coconut Blinis with Spiced Fruit Compote

Makes: 8 blinis

Preparation time: 15 minutes

Cooking time: 20 minutes

8 plums, cut into quarters, or
    400g/14oz/3¼ cups berries

3 star anise

2 cinnamon sticks

zest and juice of 1 orange

4 eggs

120ml/4fl oz/½ cup almond milk, coconut
    milk or kefir (pages 40, 41, 44)

1 tsp vanilla extract

1 tbsp maple syrup, coconut
    syrup or honey

60g/2¼oz/½ cup coconut flour

1 tsp bicarbonate of soda/baking soda

½ tsp gluten-free baking powder

1 tbsp lemon juice

a pinch of sea salt

1 tbsp coconut oil , melted, or butter or
    light olive oil, plus extra for frying

yogurt, coconut yogurt or nut
    yogurt (pages 46, 47), to serve

These little pancakes are ideal as a snack or breakfast option, and both the blinis and compote can be made in advance – simply warm them up when required. While coconut flour is high FODMAP, you could make the blinis with gluten-free flour (you will need double the amount of flour) and serve them with banana or blueberries instead of the compote.

1   To make the compote, put the plums in a pan over a medium heat with the spices and orange zest and juice. Cover and simmer gently for 5 minutes or until the fruit is just soft but holding its shape. (This can be prepared a day ahead and kept in the fridge to allow the flavours to develop.)

2   Put the remaining ingredients into a blender or food processor and blend until smooth. Heat a frying pan over a medium-low heat. Add a little coconut oil to grease the pan.

3   Ladle a tablespoonful of the batter into the pan for each blini. Cook for 2–3 minutes until the sides and base turn golden. Flip and cook for another 2 minutes. Remove from the pan and repeat with the remaining batter to make 8 blinis. Serve hot with the fruit compote. If making ahead, store the blinis in the fridge for up to 2 days.

Gut Benefits

The grain-free, low-allergen ingredients in this dish make it easy to digest. Serving it with the compote ensures you have plenty of fibre to support your digestive function, and serving it with yogurt ensures you also have some beneficial bacteria.

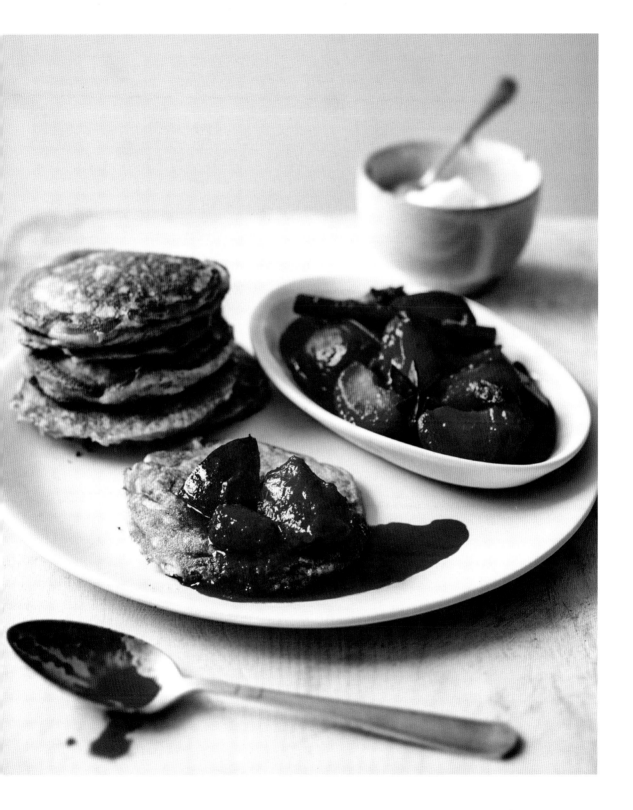

NUTRITIONAL INFORMATION PER WAFFLE   Kcals 386, Protein 9.8g, Carbs 63g of which sugars 13g, Fat 10g of which saturates 5g, Fibre 2.7g

Buttermilk Waffles with Berries

Makes: 4 waffles

Preparation time: 10 minutes

Cooking time: 12 minutes

240g/8½oz/2 cups plain
    gluten-free flour blend

2 tsp ground flaxseed

30g/1oz/2 tbsp caster sugar
    or maple syrup

1 tsp baking powder

½ tsp bicarbonate of soda

½ tsp xanthum gum

a pinch of salt

400g/14oz/1¾ cups buttermilk or kefir

2 eggs

2 tbsp melted butter

1 tsp vanilla extract

Light and crispy, these waffles make an ideal weekend breakfast. Gluten-free flour tends to be low in fibre, so I often add chia seeds or flaxseeds to increase the fibre content. You can make your own buttermilk by adding 1–2 tablespoons of lemon juice to full fat milk and leaving it to stand at room temperature for about 10 minutes. As homemade buttermilk is likely to be thinner than commercial buttermilk, you may need to reduce the amount you use in this recipe. For low FODMAP use lactose-free milk.

1   Place all the ingredients in a food processor or blender and process until smooth and creamy. Let the mixture stand for 5 minutes while you heat up the waffle iron.

2   Grease your waffle iron with a little butter or light olive oil. When the waffle iron is hot, pour in some of the batter and spread out evenly. Cook according to the manufacturer's instructions. Repeat with the remaining batter to make 4 waffles. Serve with yogurt and berries.

NUTRITIONAL INFORMATION PER SERVING Kcals 154, **Protein** 19.3g, **Carbs** 3.5g of which sugars 2.8g, **Fat** 7.5g of which saturates 4.7g **Fibre** 2.5g

Pan-Fried Indian-Spiced Liver

Serves: 2

Preparation time: 10 minutes

Cooking time: 9 minutes

200g/7oz chicken livers

1 tbsp olive oil

1 tsp cumin seeds

2.5cm/1in piece of root ginger, peeled and grated

1 red onion, finely chopped

60g/2¼oz/⅔ cup button mushrooms, cut into quarters

¼ tsp ground turmeric

½ tsp chilli powder

½ tsp ground coriander

1 tomato, deseeded and chopped

a pinch of sea salt

1 tbsp lime juice

1 handful of coriander/cilantro leaves

Inexpensive and rich with flavour, liver makes a good, speedy meal. Here, it is cut into bite-size pieces and tossed in spices, then pan-fried with vegetables. It's a delicious and nourishing dish – great for brunch or lunch as well as for breakfast, and can be served with homemade pickles.

1   Trim off any fatty parts and sinew from the chicken livers, then cut them into 2.5cm/1in dice. Leave to one side. Heat the oil in a frying pan over a medium heat and cook the cumin seeds for 30 seconds or until they release their aroma. Add the ginger and onion, and cook for 5 minutes or until the onion is soft.

2   Add the chicken livers and cook for 1 minute, then add the mushrooms and cook for 2 minutes. Add the spices and cook for 30 seconds, then add the tomato and salt. Stir in the lime juice and remove from the heat. Serve scattered with the coriander/cilantro leaves.

Gut Benefits

Organ meats, such as liver, are incredibly nutrient dense and wonderful for supporting gut healing. They are rich in many important vitamins and minerals (such as the vitamins A, D, E, K2, B12 and folic acid, and the minerals copper and iron). These nutrients also support the cleansing of toxins.

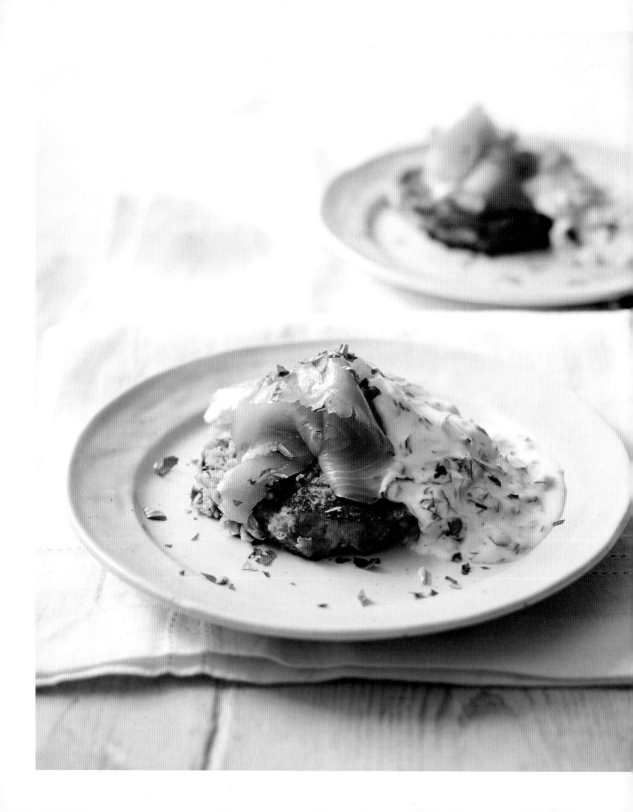

NUTRITIONAL INFORMATION PER SERVING   Kcals 398, **Protein** 23.5g, **Carbs** 26.7g of which sugars 12g, **Fat** 21.8g of which saturates 7.1g **Fibre** 5.3g

Smoked Salmon with Sweet Potato Apple Rösti

Serves: 2

Preparation time: 15 minutes

Cooking time: 15 minutes

1 sweet potato, about 200g/7oz,
    unpeeled, cut in half lengthways

1 eating apple

1 egg, beaten

2 tbsp almond flour or very finely
    ground almonds, or gluten-free
    flour, plus extra if needed

1 tbsp olive oil or ghee (page 38)

2 large slices of smoked salmon

sea salt and ground black pepper

HERBED YOGURT

60g/2¼oz/¼ cup coconut yogurt
    or yogurt (pages 47, 46)

1 tbsp chopped coriander/cilantro leaves

1 tbsp chopped mint leaves

1 tsp lemon juice

A herbed yogurt is served here with rösti and salmon. Sweet potato is a tasty and nutrient-rich alternative to potatoes, and it is exceptionally tasty combined with apple.

1   Preheat the oven to 180°C/350°F/Gas 4. To make the herbed yogurt, put the yogurt in a bowl and stir in the herbs and lemon juice. Season with salt and pepper. To make the rösti, microwave half the potato at full power for 2–3 minutes until soft. Leave to cool, then peel off the skin. (Alternatively, bake in an oven preheated to 180°C/350°F/Gas 4 for 1 hour.)

2   Mash the potato in a bowl. Coarsely grate the remaining potato and the apple onto paper towels and squeeze to remove the excess moisture. Tip into the bowl and add the egg and almond flour. Season and stir. The mixture should hold its shape. Add more almond flour if needed.

3   Heat the oil in an ovenproof frying pan over a medium heat. Divide the mixture in half and shape into 2 patties 1cm/½in thick. Use a large spatula to lift the patties into the pan. Lower the heat and cook for 2–3 minutes until the base is golden. Turn the rösti over and cook for 2–3 minutes until golden. Transfer the pan to the oven for 5 minutes to cook the rösti through. Serve topped with the salmon and a spoonful of herbed yogurt.

Gut Benefits

Nutritious sweet potato is packed with soluble fibre to support healthy gut bacteria, plus it contains gut-protective carotenoids.

NUTRITIONAL INFORMATION PER SERVING   Kcals 195, Protein 12.8g, Carbs 0.4g of which sugars 0.4g, Fat 15.8g of which saturates 7.1g Fibre 0.5g

Spiced Omelette

Serves: 2

Preparation time: 5 minutes

Cooking time: 3 minutes

4 eggs

1 tsp mirin or rice wine vinegar

¼ tsp ground turmeric or 1cm/½in
piece of turmeric root, grated

1 tsp fish sauce

2 tsp lime juice

1 tbsp chopped coriander/cilantro
leaves, plus extra to serve

1 tbsp olive oil

2 spring onions/scallions (green parts
only for low FODMAP), chopped

sea salt and ground black pepper

fermented vegetables, such as kimchi
or sauerkraut (pages 54, 52)
and ½ lime (optional), to serve

The delicate spicing of this dish combined with the fresh taste of the herbs makes this just right for breakfast. For a low FODMAP option, use the green parts of the spring onions only. Serve the omelette with fermented pickles or sauerkraut, if you like. For a vegetarian option, simply omit the fish sauce.

1   Put the eggs in a bowl and beat them. Stir in the mirin, turmeric, fish sauce, lime juice and coriander/cilantro. Season with salt and pepper to taste.

2   Heat the coconut oil in a frying pan or wok over a medium heat and cook the spring onions/scallions for 1 minute. Pour in the eggs and swirl them around the pan. Leave the eggs to cook for 1 minute, then flip over the omelette and briefly cook the other side.

3   Fold the omelette in half and cut it in half. Top with chopped coriander/cilantro and serve with fermented vegetables and a squeeze of lime, if you like.

Gut Benefits

Adding turmeric to this omelette boosts its anti-inflammatory qualities, and turmeric is also traditionally used as a carminative (to prevent gas) and a liver-supporting herb. The protein in the eggs is beneficial for gut healing.

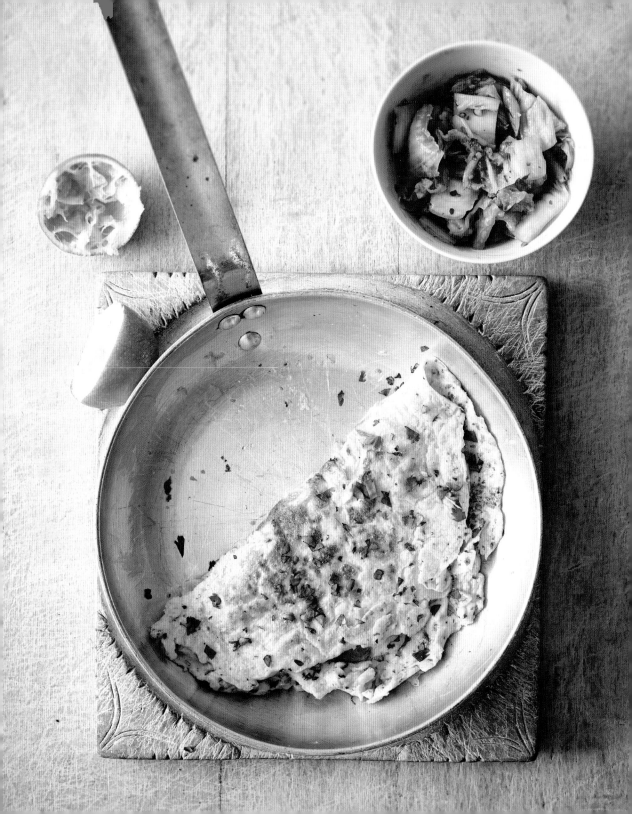

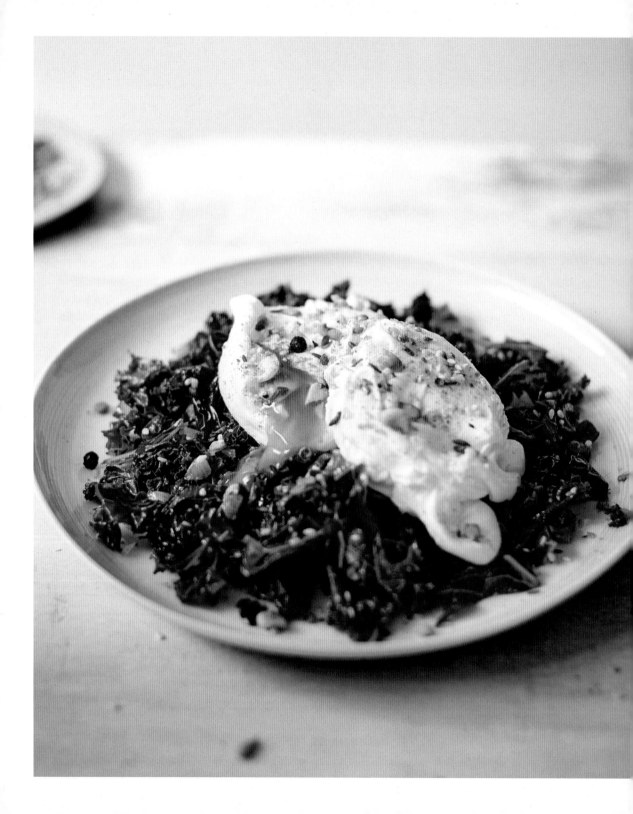

5-STEP
REM **REPL** REPA

DIETARY
| D | G | **GR** | P | S | **V** |

NUTRITIONAL INFORMATION PER SERVING   Kcals 437, Protein 19.1g, Carbs 3.8g of which sugars 2.3g, Fat 40.5g of which saturates 9g Fibre 8.7g

Poached Eggs with Wilted Kale, Tomato & Dukka

Serves: 2

Preparation time: 15 minutes

Cooking time: 15 minutes

100g/3½oz kale, chopped

2 tsp coconut oil or olive oil

1 shallot, chopped

1 garlic clove, crushed

60g/2¼oz/heaped ⅓ cup sun-dried
   tomatoes in oil, drained and chopped

4 eggs

DUKKA

50g/1¾oz/⅓ cup hazelnuts

50g/1¾oz/⅓ cup sesame seeds

1 tbsp sunflower seeds

3 tbsp coriander seeds

1 tsp peppercorns

2 tbsp cumin seeds

1 tsp smoked paprika

2 tsp sea salt

Start off the day with this hearty breakfast bowl made with dukka – an Egyptian condiment. Use the leftover dukka to flavour meat and fish dishes – it will store for up to 2 weeks.

1   To make the dukka, toast the hazelnuts in a dry frying pan over a medium heat for 1 minute or until lightly golden, stirring. Remove from the pan and leave to one side. Add the remaining ingredients and stir for 1–2 minutes to lightly toast the seeds. Put the nuts and seeds into a high-speed blender or food processor and pulse to chop the nuts, leaving texture.

2   Put the kale in a steamer and steam over a high heat for 1 minute to blanch it. Drain well. Heat the oil in a frying pan over a medium heat and cook the kale for 5 minutes or until it is slightly crispy. Add the shallot, garlic and tomatoes, and stir for another 5 minutes or until the shallot is soft. Scatter over 1 tablespoon of the dukka and mix together lightly.

3   Meanwhile, pour boiling water to a depth of 2.5cm/1in into a small frying pan over a high heat. Bring to the boil and then reduce the heat to a simmer. Crack each egg into the pan, keeping them spaced apart. Poach the eggs for 3–4 minutes until cooked to your liking. Using a slotted spoon, lift the eggs out and put them on paper towels to drain. Serve the eggs on the kale and scatter 1 tablespoon of the dukka over each.

Gut Benefits

Kale contains a number of minerals such as calcium, magnesium and potassium as well as soluble fibre to aid digestive health. The dish is also rich in zinc from the seeds, which is an important mineral for supporting digestive secretions.

NUTRITIONAL INFORMATION PER SERVING Kcals 342l, **Protein** 13g, **Carbs** 42g of which sugars 7.9g, **Fat** 12g of which saturates 1.7g, **Fibre** 7g

Overnight Oats with Kiwi & Pomegranate

Serves: 2

Preparation time: 5 minutes

Chilling: overnight

100g/3½oz jumbo oats (gluten-
free for gluten-free version)

2 tbsp mixed seeds

milk of choice

¼ tsp ground cinnamon

1–2 tbsp yogurt of choice to top

seeds from ½ pomegranate

2 kiwi fruit, chopped

This is an easy recipe to prepare ahead and a great source of soluble fibre to support bowel motility. Oats are rich in a type of soluble fibre called beta-glucan, which acts as a prebiotic providing food for beneficial bacteria in the gut.

1   Place the oats and mixed seeds in a bowl and pour over just enough milk to cover them. Stir and place in the fridge overnight.

2   In the morning stir the mixture well, adding a little more milk if it is too thick. Stir a little cinnamon through the mixture if you like.

3   Divide the oat mixture between two bowls. Top with pomegranate seeds and kiwi fruit and a spoonful of yogurt.

Gut Benefits

Kiwi fruit is great for gut health due to its high fibre content and unique enzyme, actinidin. The fibre in kiwi aids digestion and promotes regular bowel movements, which can prevent constipation. It is also a prebiotic, promoting the growth of beneficial bacteria in the gut.

NUTRITIONAL INFORMATION PER SERVING Kcals 213, Protein 17g, Carbs 7g of which sugars 3.6g, Fat 12g of which saturates 1.8g, Fibre 2.9g

Tofu Scramble

Serves: 2

Preparation time: 5 minutes

Cooking time: 6–7 minutes

2 tsp olive oil

2 spring onions/scallions (for low FODMAP, just use the top green part), sliced (optional)

150g/5½oz/1 heaped cup cherry tomatoes, halved

2 large handfuls baby spinach leaves

300g/10½oz firm tofu

2 tsp tamari soy sauce

a pinch of turmeric powder

1 tbsp nutritional yeast flakes

black pepper, to taste

A popular vegan staple for breakfast, this tofu scramble is a great source of plant-based protein. The addition of vegetables provides extra fibre and antioxidants. You can serve it on its own or with toasted bread or gluten-free bread. This recipe works equally well as a quick lunch option.

1 Heat the olive oil in a small frying pan. Add the spring onions/scallions and sauté for a couple of minutes to soften. Add the tomatoes and spinach and cook until softened for another 2 minutes.

2 Add the drained tofu. Use a spatula to break it down as much as you like, leaving some bits bigger. Allow the tofu to cook on a low heat until the excess water has cooked out.

3 Season with soy sauce, nutritional yeast, turmeric and black pepper, and gently stir through.

4 Serve on its own or with toasted bread or gluten-free bread.

Gut Benefits

Tofu is a great plant-based protein option, especially if you are following a low-FODMAP diet. It is a good source of minerals, including magnesium, iron, manganese, copper and zinc. Some varieties are also high in calcium.

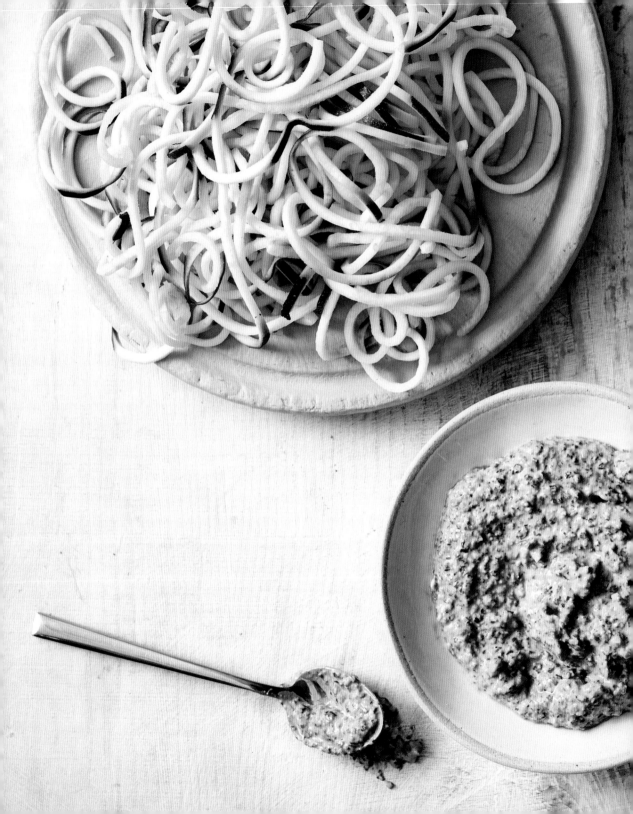

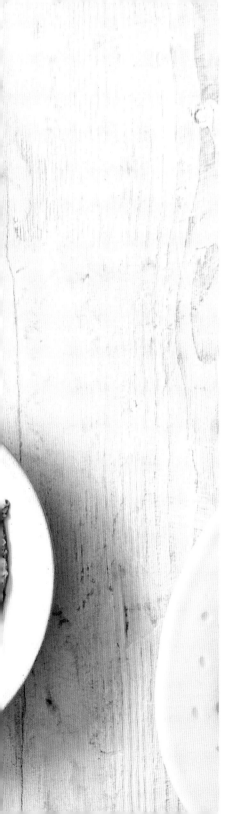

Lunches

Whether you're looking for lunch at home or something to pile into a lunch box, you'll find a great selection of healthy recipes in this chapter. From light, refreshing soups, such as my Broccoli & Watercress Cleanse, and low-carb, protein-rich salads to more comforting Paleo and grain-free options, including a delicious Broccoli Pizza and Hot-Smoked Trout with Pistachio Pesto Noodles. All the dishes are packed with nutrients designed to nourish and heal the digestive tract, using minimum effort for preparation.

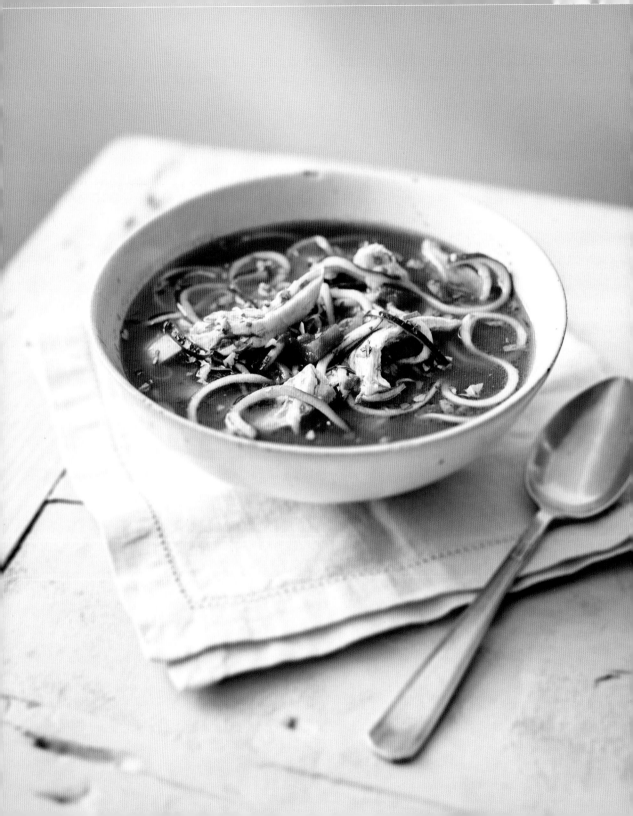

NUTRITIONAL INFORMATION PER SERVING   Kcals 165, **Protein** 27.3g, **Carbs** 6.1g of which sugars 5.8g, **Fat** 3.5g of which saturates 1.7g **Fibre** 3.7g

Restorative Chicken Noodle Soup

Serves: 2

Preparation time: 15 minutes

Cooking time: 30 minutes

2 skinless, boneless chicken breasts

400ml/14fl oz/generous 1½ cups
    chicken bone broth (page 37)

1 tsp olive oil

2 spring onions/scallions (green parts
    only for low FODMAP), sliced

1 celery stalk, diced

½ red chilli, deseeded and diced

1 garlic clove, crushed (optional)

200g/7oz/scant 3¾ cup canned
    chopped tomatoes

½ red pepper/bell pepper,
    deseeded and diced

1 tsp tomato purée/paste

a pinch of smoked paprika

½ tsp ground cumin

1 courgette/zucchini, about 150g/5½oz

1 handful of coriander/cilantro
    leaves, chopped

sea salt and ground black pepper

This low-carb healing soup uses strips of courgette/zucchini instead of regular noodles. You can make this low FODMAP by leaving out the garlic and using only the green tops of the spring onions/scallions. For a more hearty option replace the courgette with rice noodles or buckwheat noodles.

1   Put the chicken breasts in a saucepan over a medium-high heat and pour over the broth. Bring to the boil, then reduce the heat and simmer for 15 minutes. Turn off the heat and leave the chicken to continue cooking in the stock for a further 5 minutes or until cooked through. Remove the chicken from the broth and leave to one side. Reserve the broth.

2   Heat the coconut oil in large saucepan and cook the spring onions/scallions, celery, chilli and garlic, if using, for 2–3 minutes until the celery is soft. Add the tomatoes and reserved broth, and add the red pepper/bell pepper, tomato purée/paste and spices. Cook over a low heat for 5 minutes or until the vegetables are soft.

3   Use a spiralizer to create courgette/zucchini noodles, or use a sharp knife to cut the courgette/zucchini lengthways into thin slices and then into thin strips. Shred the chicken and add it to the pan followed by the noodles. Simmer for 1–2 minutes until the courgette/zucchini noodles are just soft. Season to taste and serve topped with coriander/cilantro.

Gut Benefits

Garlic is a potent antimicrobial food that is useful for tackling gut infections but it is also a high fructan food, which is why it is not suitable for a low FODMAP diet. Use garlic-infused oil instead for flavour. The antioxidant-rich ingredients make this a nourishing soup for lowering inflammation and supporting healing.

NUTRITIONAL INFORMATION PER SERVING Kcals 183, **Protein** 5.4g, **Carbs** 17.7g of which sugars 16.8g, **Fat** 10.1g of which saturates 1.6g **Fibre** 4.5g

Spiced Roasted Beetroot & Apple Soup

Serves: 2

Preparation time: 15 minutes

Cooking time: 45 minutes

250g/9oz beetroot/beet, diced

1 eating apple, cored and cut into quarters

½ onion, cut into quarters

1 garlic clove, peeled and left whole

2 tbsp olive oil

1 tsp cumin seeds

½ tsp ground coriander

½ tsp ground cinnamon

a pinch of ground ginger

zest and juice of 1 lime

500ml/17fl oz/2 cups chicken or
   beef bone broth (page 37)

leaves from 2 mint sprigs, finely
   chopped, plus extra leaves to serve

100g/3½oz/heaped ⅓ cup coconut
   yogurt or yogurt (pages 46, 47)

sea salt and ground black pepper

Roasting the beetroot and apple intensifies the flavour and creates a wonderfully sweet caramel-like hint to this rustic soup. Serve topped with yogurt. For a vegetarian or vegan option, use vegetable stock instead of bone broth.

1   Preheat the oven to 200°C/400°F/Gas 6. Put the beetroot/beet in a bowl and add the apple, onion and garlic. Drizzle in the oil and toss to mix well. Tip into a roasting pan. Season with salt and pepper, and roast for 35 minutes or until tender.

2   Lightly toast the cumin seeds in a dry saucepan over a medium heat for 30 seconds, stirring. Put the roasted vegetables into a blender or food processor with the cumin seeds and the remaining ingredients, except the mint and yogurt, and blend until smooth. Pour into a saucepan and heat over a medium-high heat until simmering. Cook for 5 minutes. Stir the mint into the yogurt. Serve the soup topped with a spoonful of the minty yogurt and scattered with mint leaves.

Gut Benefits

Beetroots/beets are known for their ability to support bile flow, making it easier to digest and absorb fats in the diet. They are also ideal for cleansing the body. Apples contain soluble and insoluble fibre to help food to move through your digestive tract more quickly for healthy elimination.

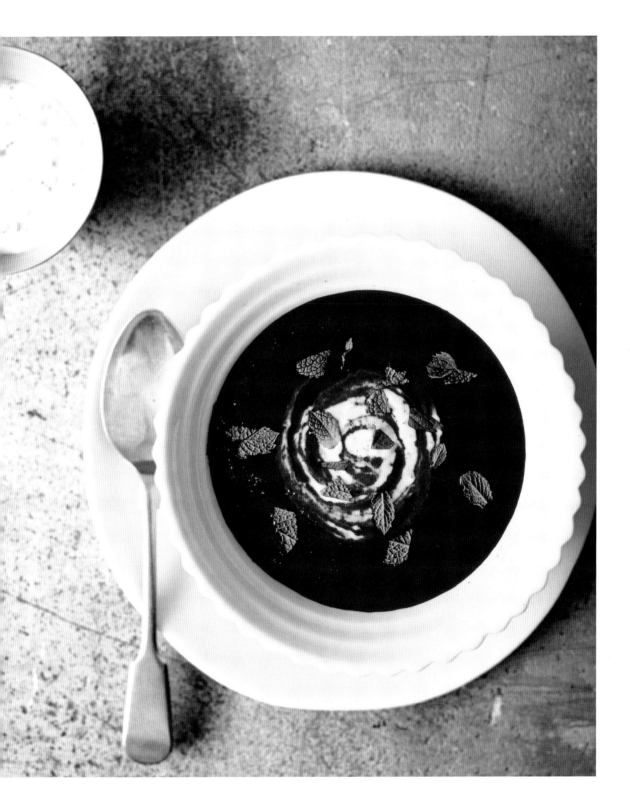

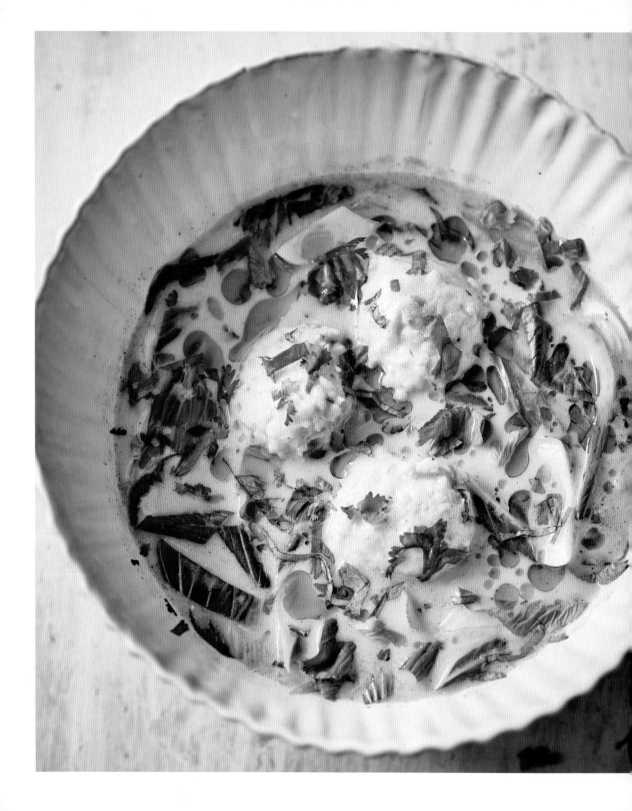

NUTRITIONAL INFORMATION PER SERVING Kcals 171, **Protein** 21.6g, **Carbs** 12.3g of which sugars 10.5g, **Fat** 3.9g of which saturates 0.8g **Fibre** 1.8g

Asian Coconut Broth with Prawn Dumplings

Serves: 2

Preparation time: 15 minutes

Cooking time: 10 minutes

400ml/14fl oz/generous 1½ cups
   full-fat canned coconut milk

100ml/3½fl oz/generous ⅓ cup
   chicken bone broth (page 37)

1–2 tsp tom yum paste, to taste

¼ tsp ground turmeric

1 spring onion/scallion, finely sliced

1 tsp tamari soy sauce or coconut aminos

100g/3½oz baby spinach leaves or
   pak choi/bok choy, shredded

1 handful of coriander/cilantro
   leaves, chopped

1 tsp sesame oil

PRAWN DUMPLINGS

200g/7oz shelled raw prawns/
   shrimp or white fish

5mm/¼in piece of root ginger,
   peeled and grated

1 spring onion/scallion, chopped

1 egg white

1 tsp arrowroot or cornflour/cornstarch

 sea salt and ground black pepper

Homemade broth and coconut milk make this a light and healing dish. The prawn dumplings can also be made with minced beef. Instead of arrowroot, use cornflour, if tolerated.

1 To make the dumplings, put the prawns/shrimp into a food processor and add the ginger and spring onion/scallion. Process until finely chopped. Add the egg white and arrowroot, and season with salt and pepper. Process to combine, then form into 4–6 balls.

2 Heat the coconut milk and broth in a saucepan over a medium-high heat until boiling. Reduce the heat and add the tom yum paste, turmeric, spring onion/scallion and tamari, then simmer gently for 3 minutes.

3 Drop in the dumplings and spinach. Cook for 3–4 minutes until the balls rise to the surface. Spoon into bowls and top with the coriander/cilantro leaves and a drizzle of sesame oil, then serve.

Gut Benefits

Bone broth is a powerful gut-healing food that is rich in valuable minerals. The amino acids in bone broth may also support a healthy gut barrier. Prawns/shrimp provide essential protein and anti-inflammatory omega-3 fats and vitamin E, which has gut- and liver-protective antioxidant benefits.

NUTRITIONAL INFORMATION PER SERVING   Kcals 180, Protein 10.1g, Carbs 7.6g of which sugars 4.6g, Fat 12.1g of which saturates 4.3g Fibre 8.3g

Broccoli & Watercress Cleanse

Serves: 2

Preparation time: 10 minutes

Cooking time: 15 minutes

2 tsp olive oil

1 garlic clove, chopped

1 onion, chopped

300g/10½oz broccoli, broken into florets

500ml/17fl oz/2 cups vegetable stock
   or chicken bone broth (page 37)

1 large handful of watercress

1 tbsp lemon juice

30g/1oz/¼ cup cashew nuts

sea salt and ground black pepper

Light and refreshing, this soup uses cruciferous vegetables, which have strong cleansing properties. The addition of a few nuts gives it a creamier texture and provides a little protein, but you could use a spoonful of homemade yogurt instead.

1   Heat the coconut oil in a saucepan over a medium heat. Add the garlic and onion, and cook for 1–2 minutes until just beginning to soften. Add the broccoli and cook for 3–4 minutes, making sure it is coated in the oil.

2   Pour in the stock and season with salt and pepper. Bring to the boil, then lower the heat. Cover and simmer for 6–7 minutes until the broccoli is just tender. Pour the soup into a blender or food processor and add the watercress, lemon juice and cashews, then blend until smooth. Return to the pan and reheat gently before serving.

Gut Benefits

Cruciferous vegetables are rich in glucosinolates known for their anti-cancer, anti-inflammatory and detoxification benefits. They also contain calcium D-glucarate, which can be helpful for lowering high levels of beta glucuronidase which is involved in the recirculation of oestrogen.

NUTRITIONAL INFORMATION PER SERVING   Kcals 436, Protein 26.7g, Carbs 6g of which sugars 5g, Fat 33.7g of which saturates 5g Fibre 3.8g

Chicken & Artichoke Salad with Roasted Garlic & Herb Dressing

Serves: 2

Preparation time: 15 minutes, plus
   cooling

Cooking time: 30 minutes

2 skinless, boneless chicken breasts

1 cos or romaine lettuce, shredded

1 handful of rocket/arugula leaves

2 marinated artichoke hearts,
   drained and quartered

1 handful of pitted black olives, sliced

½ red onion, thinly sliced

100g/3½oz/heaped ⅔ cup cherry
   tomatoes, cut into halves

GARLIC AND HERB DRESSING

2 garlic cloves, unpeeled

60ml/2fl oz/¼ cup olive oil,
   plus extra to drizzle

¼ tsp Dijon mustard, or to taste

1 tbsp chopped parsley leaves

1 tbsp red wine vinegar

1 tbsp sherry vinegar

½ tsp sugar, or to taste

sea salt and ground black pepper

You can prepare this Mediterranean-inspired salad in the morning and add the dressing just before serving. It's good served with homemade sauerkraut.

1   Preheat the oven to 200°C/400°F/Gas 6. To make the dressing, put the garlic cloves on a piece of foil, drizzle over a little oil and wrap up the foil. Cook in the oven for 30 minutes or until soft. Leave to cool.

2   Meanwhile, bring a large saucepan of water to the boil. Add the chicken breasts and simmer for 10 minutes. Turn off the heat and leave the chicken to stand in the water for 15 minutes or until the chicken is cooked through. Remove from the water.

3   Squeeze out the flesh of the cooled garlic into a blender or a mini food processor and add the remaining dressing ingredients. Process until smooth.

4   Shred the chicken. Put all the remaining salad ingredients in a large bowl and scatter over the chicken. Just before serving, pour over the dressing and toss well. The dressing will keep in the fridge for up to 2 days.

Gut Benefits

Globe artichokes are a popular prebiotic, providing food for the friendly bacteria that inhabit the digestive system. Just one handful of bitter greens, such as rocket/arugula or watercress, added to a salad will aid the secretion of digestive juices.

NUTRITIONAL INFORMATION PER SERVING   Kcals 235, Protein 20.2g, Carbs 10g of which sugars 7.7g, Fat 13.1g of which saturates 6.2g Fibre 3.2g

Asian-Spiced Lettuce Wraps

Serves: 2

Preparation time: 15 minutes

Cooking time: 15 minutes

2 tsp olive oil

200g/7oz minced/ground pork

1 shallot, finely chopped

½ red pepper/bell pepper,
   deseeded and diced

100g/3½oz pineapple, diced

1 large handful of basil leaves, chopped

1 large handful of mint leaves, chopped

1 large handful of coriander/cilantro
   leaves, chopped

Little Gem/Bibb lettuce, leaves separated

LIME AND CHILLI DRESSING

juice of 2 limes

1 tsp sugar

1 small garlic clove, crushed

½ red chilli, deseeded and finely chopped

1 tbsp fish sauce

2 tsp finely chopped coriander/cilantro
   leaves

As well as tasting good, serving pineapple with pork is healthy because the pineapple is a digestive aid. Spoon the pork into little lettuce leaves for a low-carb, high-protein, gut-nurturing lunch. Accompany with homemade pickles and a spoonful of homemade mayonnaise. For a vegan option you can replace the pork with crumbled tempeh or vegan mince.

1   Put the dressing ingredients in a small bowl and whisk well to combine.

2   Heat the oil in a frying pan over a medium-high heat and add the pork and shallot. Stir-fry for 10–15 minutes until the pork is brown and cooked through, breaking it up with a spoon. Add the red pepper/bell pepper, pineapple and herbs and turn off the heat. Put in a bowl and pour over the dressing. Toss well. Arrange the lettuce leaves on a plate. Spoon the pork into the lettuce leaves and serve.

Gut Benefits

Pineapple is rich in the enzyme bromelain, which is well known to support digestion and lower inflammation. Lean meats also provide a good source of B vitamins and zinc to support mood as well as gut health.

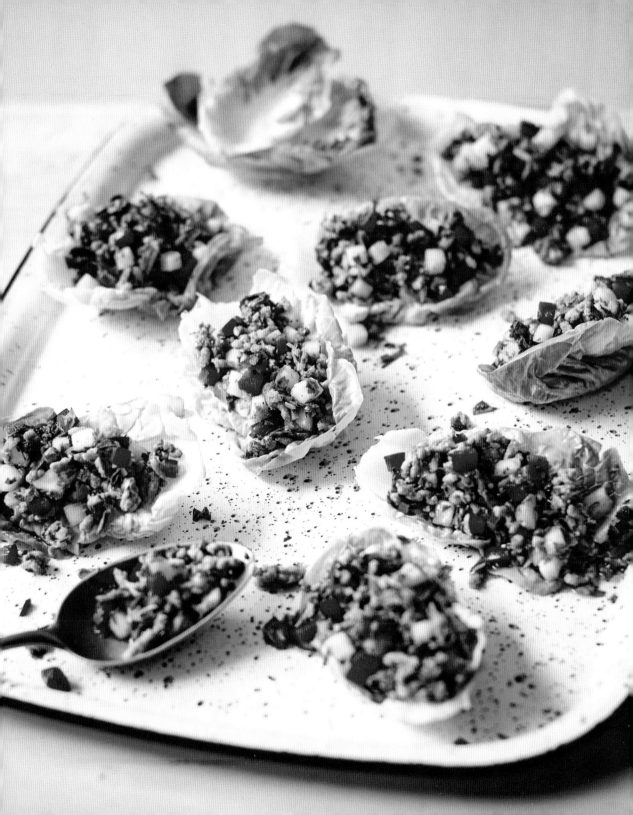

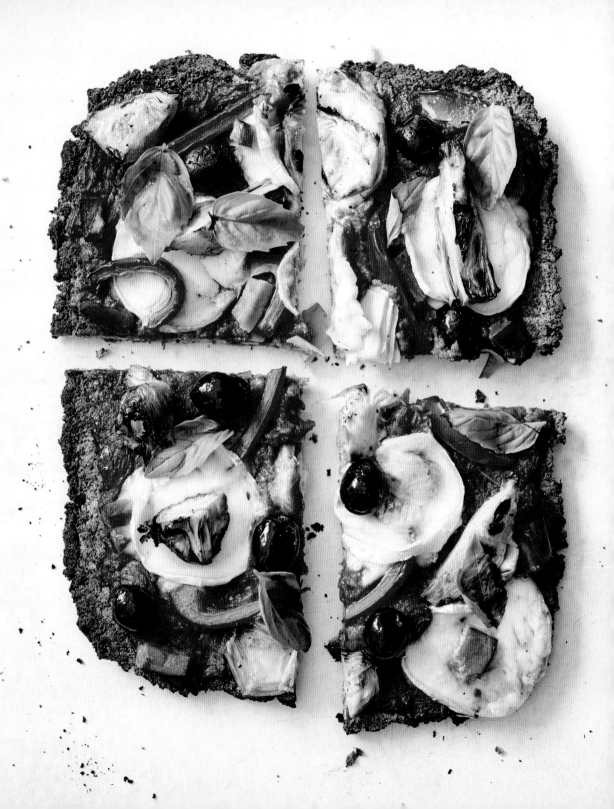

NUTRITIONAL INFORMATION PER SLICE **Kcals** 266, **Protein** 18.8g, **Carbs** 9.9g of which sugars 3.4g, **Fat** 16.5g of which saturates 7g **Fibre** 8.6g

Broccoli Pizza

Makes: 1 large pizza, 4 slices

Preparation time: 20 minutes

Cooking time: 1 hour

coconut oil or olive oil, for greasing

30g/1oz/scant ¼ cup unblanched almonds

1 small head of broccoli

30g/1oz/¼ cup coconut flour

½ tsp onion powder

½ tsp garlic salt

2 tbsp nutritional yeast flakes

2 large eggs

ground black pepper

TOPPINGS

125ml/4fl oz/½ cup ready-made
    tomato sauce or passata

a selection of vegetables such as sliced
    red pepper/bell pepper, olives, sliced
    marinated artichokes, sliced tomatoes

strips of ham or chicken, sliced cooked
    beef, cooked prawns/shrimp or other
    seafood, goat's cheese (if tolerated),
    nut cheese (page 49), herbs

Prepare this fun, low-carb, grain-free Paleo pizza as a vegetarian or meat option. Simply choose a range of toppings according to your taste. Omit the cheese for Paleo, or use goat's cheese, if tolerated, or nut cheese to make this a vegetarian pizza.

1   Preheat the oven to 190°C/375°F/Gas 5. Grease and line a baking sheet with baking parchment, then lightly oil the baking parchment. Put the almonds into a high-speed blender or food processor and process until very fine. Transfer to a bowl and leave to one side.

2   Put the broccoli into the food processor and pulse to form little rice-like pieces. Put in a bowl and microwave for 4 minutes on full power, or dry-fry in a frying pan, covered, for 2 minutes or until just soft.

3   Put all the remaining ingredients in the food processor, followed by the almonds, and process until smooth. Add the broccoli and briefly process to combine thoroughly.

4   Spread the dough on the prepared baking sheet and, using your hands, shape it into a circle or rectangle to form a 1cm/½in-thick layer. Bake the pizza base for 30–40 minutes until lightly golden.

5   Very carefully flip over the pizza base and put it back on the sheet. Bake for a further 5 minutes. Remove from the oven and spoon over the tomato sauce. Add your choice of toppings and return to the oven for 10 minutes or until cooked through. Cut into slices and serve.

Gut Benefits

Broccoli is a source of soluble fibre and provides food for beneficial bacteria. Known for its potent phytochemicals, it helps to lower inflammation and support detoxification.

NUTRITIONAL INFORMATION PER SERVING   Kcals 364, **Protein** 21.5g, **Carbs** 18.6g of which sugars 15.6g, **Fat** 26.8g of which saturates 9.1g **Fibre** 3.9g

Lebanese Lamb Salad

Serves: 2

Preparation time: 15 minutes, plus
   overnight marinating

Cooking time: 16 minutes, plus
   10 minutes resting

200–250g/7–9oz lamb loin
   or 2 lamb steaks

1 cos or romaine lettuce, cut into ribbons

100g/3½oz/heaped ⅔ cup cherry
   tomatoes, cut into halves

½ cucumber, cut in half lengthways
   and then into slices

2 radishes, sliced

½ red pepper/bell pepper, deseeded
   and cut into chunks

1 celery stalk, sliced

1 handful of mint leaves, chopped

POMEGRANATE DRESSING

2 tbsp pomegranate molasses

1 tbsp lemon juice

½ garlic clove, crushed

¼ tsp ground cumin

a pinch of stevia or sugar

2 tbsp olive oil

¼ tsp sumac powder

sea salt and ground black pepper

This Middle Eastern-style salad combines a light, refreshing lemon–pomegranate dressing with crisp vegetables and sliced lamb to make an energizing lunch. It's very good served topped with a spoonful of homemade mayonnaise, too.

1   Put the dressing ingredients in a small bowl. Season lightly and whisk well to combine.

2   Put the lamb in a shallow dish and drizzle a little of the dressing over the top. Cover and marinate overnight in the fridge.

3   Preheat the oven to 200°C/400°F/Gas 6. Heat an ovenproof frying pan over a medium-high heat until hot, then put the lamb into the pan and sear it for 2–3 minutes on each side.

4   Transfer the pan to the oven and cook for 10 minutes or until the lamb is cooked but still slightly pink in the middle. Remove from the oven and leave on a warm plate to rest for 10 minutes. Slice thinly.

5   Put the lettuce in a large serving bowl and add the tomatoes, cucumber, radishes, red pepper/bell pepper, celery and mint. Add the lamb slices and drizzle over the remaining dressing, then serve.

Gut Benefits

Grass-fed lamb is rich in CLA (conjugated linoleic acid), a health-supportive fatty acid. It also provides essential amino acids and protein as well as key nutrients, including zinc, selenium and B vitamins, for gut healing and supporting the stress hormones.

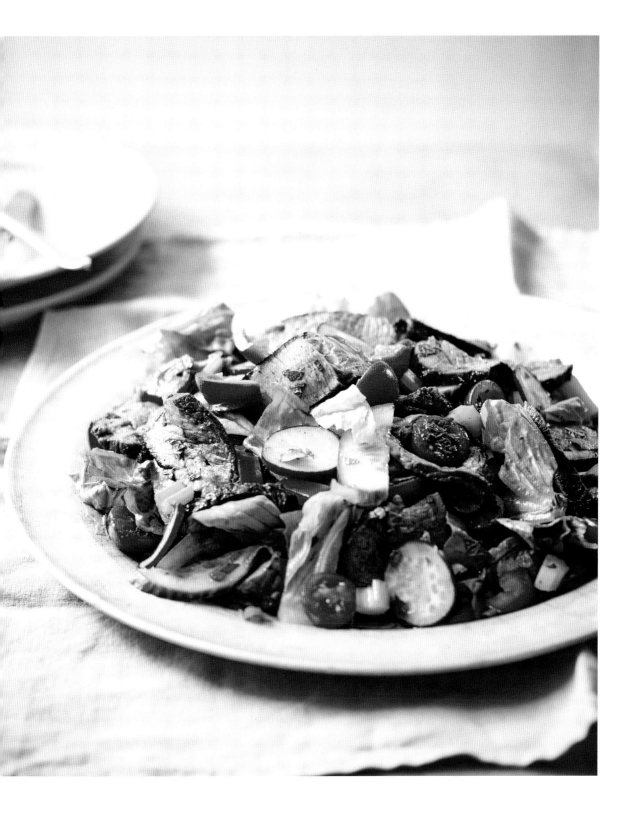

NUTRITIONAL INFORMATION PER SERVING   Kcals 234, **Protein** 29.9g, **Carbs** 14.1g of which sugars 7.5g, **Fat** 7.2g of which saturates 2.5g **Fibre** 7.1g

Purple-Sprouting Broccoli & Beef Kelp Noodle Salad

Serves: 2

Preparation time: 15 minutes, plus

   15 minutes soaking

Cooking time: 13 minutes, plus

   10 minutes resting

100g/3½oz kelp noodles

200g/7oz purple-sprouting

   broccoli, cut into short pieces

200g/7oz sirloin steak, trimmed

1 tsp fish sauce

1 tsp olive oil

1 garlic clove, crushed

2 spring onions/scallions, chopped

½ cucumber, deseeded and cut into strips

1 small carrot, cut into strips

ground black pepper

GINGER DRESSING

2 tbsp tamari soy sauce or

   coconut aminos

1 tbsp sugar

1 red chilli, deseeded and diced

1 garlic clove, crushed

5mm/¼in piece of root ginger,

   peeled and grated

juice of 1 lime

Serve this Asian-inspired salad for an energizing lunch or as a light dinner option. Purple-sprouting broccoli is at its best during the spring, so use regular broccoli if not available. You can use salmon or chicken instead of the beef, if you like. Kelp noodles are available from health food shops or online. Alternatively, use buckwheat or rice noodles.

1   Soak the kelp noodles in cold water for 15 minutes, then drain in a colander and rinse thoroughly. Put the broccoli in a steamer and steam over a high heat for 2–3 minutes until just tender but still with some bite. Transfer to a colander and refresh under cold water, then drain and leave to one side.

2   Put the dressing ingredients in a small bowl and whisk well. Put the noodles in a large bowl and pour over the dressing, mix well and leave to one side while you prepare the beef.

3   Rub the steak with the fish sauce and olive oil, and season with pepper. Heat a frying pan over a medium-high heat. Sear the steak for 3–4 minutes on each side. Remove from the pan and leave on a warm plate to rest for 5–10 minutes. Slice thinly.

4   In the same pan, add the garlic, then stir-fry the broccoli over a medium heat for 1–2 minutes until heated through. Put the broccoli in the bowl with the noodles and add the spring onions/scallions, cucumber and carrot. Toss together well. Serve the steak with the noodles.

Gut Benefits

Low-carb kelp noodles are rich in a variety of valuable minerals, including iodine, calcium, iron and vitamin K. They are also a good source of bowel-beneficial soluble fibre.

NUTRITIONAL INFORMATION PER SERVING   Kcals 339, Protein 27.4g, Carbs 12g of which sugars 5.1g, Fat 20.8g of which saturates 4.8g Fibre 3.9g

Lime-Marinated Salmon Salad with Fennel & Mango

Serves: 2

Preparation time: 20 minutes, plus
   30 minutes marinating

Cooking time: 6 minutes, plus cooling

juice of 3 limes

2 tsp sugar

½ garlic clove, crushed

1 tbsp fish sauce

2 boneless salmon fillets with skin,
   about 130g/4½oz each

1 tsp coconut oil

1 large handful of rocket/arugula leaves

½ cos or romaine lettuce, shredded

½ red onion, finely chopped

½ mango, peeled and thinly sliced

½ ripe avocado, peeled and diced

½ fennel bulb, cored and very thinly sliced

½ red chilli, deseeded and chopped

1 small handful of coriander/cilantro
   leaves, chopped

1 small handful of mint leaves,
   finely chopped

sea salt and ground black pepper

Salmon fillets are marinated in a tangy lime dressing before cooking, making this a light, refreshing dish. You could also accompany this with a spoonful of homemade beetroot sauerkraut, if you like.

1   Put the lime juice in a bowl and add the sugar, garlic and fish sauce. Season with salt and pepper, and whisk together.

2   Put the salmon fillets in a shallow dish and pour over half the dressing. Chill in the fridge for 30 minutes.

3   Heat the oil in a frying pan over a medium-high heat and add the salmon with its marinade. Cook for 3 minutes on each side until cooked through, then leave to cool. Remove the skin and flake the salmon into large pieces.

4   Put the rocket/arugula and lettuce on plates. Add the onion, mango, avocado, fennel and chilli, then top the salad with the flaked salmon. Scatter over the chopped herbs and serve with the remaining dressing.

Gut Benefits

Salmon, like other oily fish, contains essential anti-inflammatory omega-3 fats, which are ideal for gut healing and supporting brain health. Fennel bulb is known for its digestive benefits. It is rich in soluble fibre and the essential oil anethole, which helps to lower inflammation and relieve gut spasms.

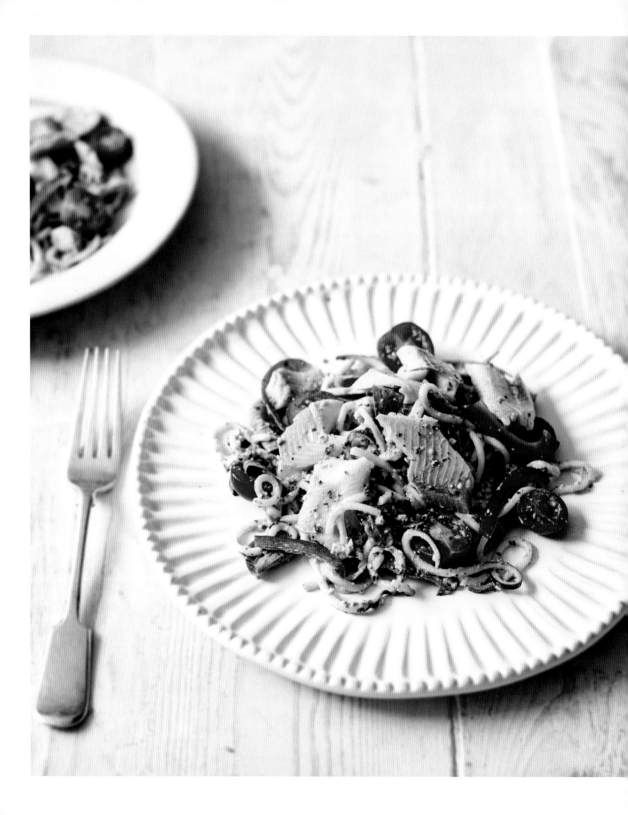

NUTRITIONAL INFORMATION PER SERVING   Kcals 364, **Protein** 36.2g, **Carbs** 6.2g of which sugars 5g, **Fat** 21.7g of which saturates 6.7g **Fibre** 3.6g

Hot-Smoked Trout with Pistachio Pesto Noodles

Serves: 2

Preparation time: 15 minutes

30g/1oz/¼ cup pistachio nuts

1 garlic clove, crushed

a pinch of sea salt

2 handfuls of basil leaves

60g/2¼oz/¼ cup coconut yogurt
    or yogurt (pages 47, 46),
    plus extra if needed

1 tsp olive oil

2 tsp lemon juice

2 small courgettes/zucchini

2 handfuls of baby spinach leaves

80–100g (or 8) cherry
    tomatoes, cut into halves

¼ red pepper/bell pepper,
    deseeded and cut into strips

2 hot-smoked trout fillets, about
    130g/4½oz each, broken into pieces

Baby spinach leaves and courgette/zucchini noodles are tossed with a creamy, nutty and protein-rich pesto and topped with flaked hot-smoked trout for this flavourful dish. Adding a little yogurt to the pesto is a great way to include some beneficial bacteria. For a vegetarian option, omit the trout and scatter over a spoonful of toasted seeds and chopped hard-boiled egg or pan-fried chunks of tofu.

1   Put the pistachios into a high-speed blender or mini food processor and add the garlic and salt. Blend until the nuts are finely ground. Add the basil leaves, coconut yogurt, oil and lemon juice, and blend until well combined. Add a little more yogurt if needed to create a smooth, thick dressing.

2   Use a spiralizer to create courgette/zucchini noodles, or a swivel vegetable peeler to make thin ribbons. Put the noodles in a large bowl and add the spinach leaves.

3   Add the pesto dressing and toss well to combine. Serve topped with the cherry tomatoes, red pepper/bell pepper and trout fillets.

Gut Benefits

This low-carb, grain-free dish is rich in probiotic bacteria from the yogurt and contains antioxidant-rich veggies. Pistachio nuts contain polyphenolic antioxidant compounds, which promote the growth of beneficial gut flora, and minerals, including zinc, to support digestion and aid gut healing. Oily fish, such as trout, contain plenty of anti-inflammatory omega-3 fats.

NUTRITIONAL INFORMATION PER SERVING   Kcals 389, Protein 23.3g, Carbs 24.5g of which sugars 0.1g, Fat 22.4g of which saturates 4.4g Fibre 1.5g

Tamarind-Glazed Mackerel

Serves: 2

Preparation time: 10 minutes, plus

30 minutes marinating

Cooking time: 10 minutes

Tangy and sweet, tamarind makes a delicious sauce to serve with mackerel or other oily fish. Accompany with homemade sauerkraut or pickles for a speedy lunch. Add a spoonful of homemade mayonnaise, if you like.

70g/2½oz/3 heaped tbsp tamarind paste

1 tbsp of sugar

½ tsp ground cumin

2 tsp lemon juice

5mm/¼in piece of root ginger,
   peeled and grated

2 small mackerel, boned, cleaned
   and heads removed

2 tsp olive oil, plus extra for greasing

sea salt

steamed pak choi/bok choy
   and sauerkraut or kimchi
   (pages 52, 54), to serve

1   Put the tamarind paste in a bowl and add 1 tablespoon water, the sugar, cumin, lemon juice and ginger.

2   Score the mackerel fillets twice on each side, then lay them in a shallow dish. Spoon half the tamarind mixture over the mackerel fillets and leave them in the fridge to marinate for 30 minutes. Put the remaining sauce in a small serving bowl.

3   Preheat the grill/broiler and grease a baking sheet. Put the mackerel on the prepared baking sheet, skin-side up. Sprinkle the fillets with the olive oil and some sea salt, then grill/broil them for 5 minutes on each side or until the flesh is opaque and cooked through. Serve the mackerel with pak choi/bok choy and sauerkraut and the remaining tamarind sauce.

Gut Benefits

Tangy tamarind has long been used for easing stomach discomfort, aiding digestion and as a laxative. Mackerel provides anti-inflammatory omega-3 fats and vitamin D – known for its role in promoting digestive health and gut repair.

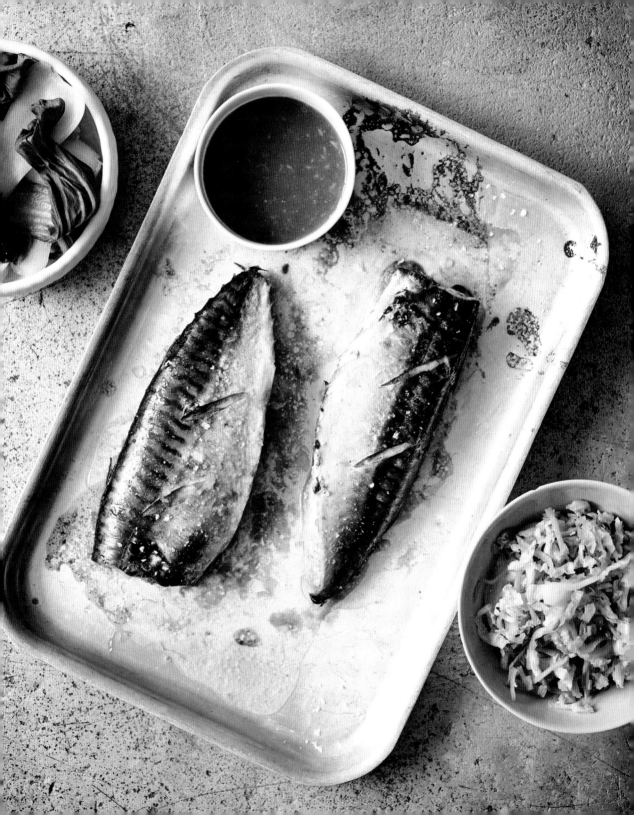

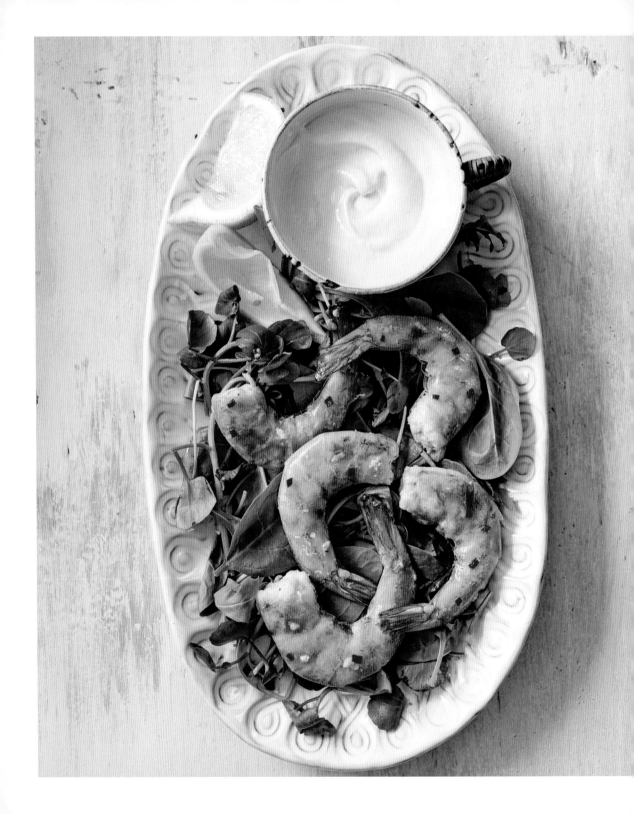

NUTRITIONAL INFORMATION PER SERVING WITH 2 TABLESPOONS AIOLI   Kcals 387, Protein 22.6g, Carbs 0.2g of which sugars 0g, Fat 32.8g of which saturates 7.6g Fibre 0.6g

Grilled Prawns with Turmeric Lemon Aioli

Serves: 2

Preparation time: 20 minutes

Cooking time: 3 minutes

300g/10½oz shell-on raw king
   prawns/jumbo shrimp

1 tbsp coconut oil, olive oil or
   ghee (page 38), melted

1 garlic clove, crushed

1 tsp lemon juice

½ red chilli, deseeded and diced

sea salt and ground black pepper

salad leaves/greens and lemon
   wedges, to serve

TURMERIC LEMON AIOLI

½ garlic clove, crushed

½ tsp sea salt

¼ tsp ground turmeric

½ tsp lemon zest

1 egg yolk

100ml/3½fl oz/generous ⅓ cup
   extra virgin olive oil

60ml/2fl oz/¼ cup walnut or
   macadamia nut oil

juice of ½ lemon

The tangy aioli is rich and creamy and a wonderful addition for simply grilled prawns/shrimp as well as other plainly cooked seafood and chicken. It will make a little more than you need, but it stores well in the fridge for up to 3 days and can be served with salad or vegetables and homemade sauerkraut or pickles.

1   To make the aioli, put the garlic, salt, turmeric and lemon zest in a mini food processor, or use a stick blender and beaker, and pulse to combine. Add the egg. Very slowly add the oils with the motor running, followed by the lemon juice. Process until the mixture is thick and emulsified.

2   Using a sharp serrated knife, cut each prawn/shrimp through the shell on the back just enough to remove the vein. Remove the head, if you prefer.

3   Preheat the grill/broiler. Put the prawns/shrimp in a shallow baking dish. Put the coconut oil in a bowl and add the garlic, lemon juice and chilli, then season with salt and pepper. Mix together well, then brush over the prawns/shrimp. Grill/broil for 2–3 minutes, until the prawns/shrimp are pink and just cooked. Serve the prawns/shrimp with salad, lemon wedges and 2 tablespoons of aioli for each portion.

Gut Benefits

Prawns/shrimp are a good source of the anti-inflammatory carotenoid nutrient astaxanthin, plus omega-3 fats, choline, zinc and selenium, all of which are important nutrients for protecting and healing the gut.

NUTRITIONAL INFORMATION PER SERVING   Kcals 395, Protein 9.9g, Carbs 21.4g of which sugars 12.4g, Fat 31.5g of which saturates 15.5g Fibre 1.1g

Raw Pad Thai with Courgette & Carrot Noodles

Serves: 2

Preparation time: 15 minutes

Cooking time: 1 minute

2 tbsp cashew nuts

1 carrot

1 courgette/zucchini

1 handful of baby spinach leaves

1 red pepper/bell pepper,
    deseeded and thinly sliced

40g/1½ oz/½ cup coconut flakes

1 handful of coriander/cilantro
    leaves, chopped

NUT DRESSING

2 tbsp almond nut butter

2 tsp lemon juice

1 tsp yacon syrup, coconut
    syrup or maple syrup

1 tbsp tamari soy sauce or coconut aminos

1 tbsp coconut oil, melted

½ tsp ground cumin

a pinch of chilli powder or dried
    chilli/hot pepper flakes

ground black pepper

Creamy yet light and nourishing, this is a wonderful vegan salad. It's a simple dish that is quick to prepare and it will keep in a lunch box very well. For additional protein, add pan-fried tofu or tempeh to this dish.

1   Put the dressing ingredients in a small bowl and whisk well to combine, adding enough water to create a thick sauce.

2   Lightly toast the nuts in a dry saucepan over a medium heat for 1 minute, stirring. Leave to one side.

3   Use a spiralizer to create carrot and courgette/zucchini noodles, or use a swivel vegetable peeler to make thin strips. Put the noodles in a large bowl and add the spinach leaves and red pepper/bell pepper. Pour over the nut dressing and toss well. Scatter over the nuts, coconut flakes and coriander/cilantro leaves, then serve.

Gut Benefits

This dish is easy to digest because it is low in carbs and high in soluble fibre from the vegetables. Almond nut butter is a protein-rich food, and protein is crucial for tissue regeneration and repair. There are also protective antioxidants from the vitamin E in the nut butter.

NUTRITIONAL INFORMATION PER SERVING   Kcals 444, Protein 7g, Carbs 7.2g of which sugars 6.4g, Fat 40.8g of which saturates 4.8g Fibre 3.9g

Sicilian Tabbouleh with Cauliflower Rice

Serves: 2

Preparation time: 15 minutes

Cooking time: 4 minutes

2 tbsp pine nuts

½ cauliflower, roughly chopped

1 tsp coconut oil

½ red onion, diced

½ tsp ground cumin

¼ tsp ground coriander

1 handful each of parsley, mint
   and coriander/cilantro leaves,
   roughly chopped, plus extra
   finely chopped leaves to serve

½ tsp sea salt

juice of 1 lemon

1 preserved lemon, rind only, chopped

60ml/2fl oz/¼ cup flaxseed oil or olive oil

½ cucumber, deseeded and
   finely chopped

2 plum tomatoes, deseeded
   and finely diced

2 spring onions/scallions, chopped

Lemon and lots of fresh herbs give this dish lightness and fragrance, making it taste refreshing. For additional protein, serve with some poached fish, chicken or pan-fried tofu. Top with a spoonful of homemade vegan mayonnaise, if you like.

1   Lightly toast the pine nuts in a dry saucepan over a medium heat for 1 minute, stirring, then leave to one side.

2   Put the cauliflower into a food processor or electric chopper and process into small rice-like pieces, then transfer to a large bowl and leave to one side.

3   Heat the coconut oil in a frying pan over a medium heat and cook the onion with the cumin and ground coriander for 2–3 minutes until soft.

4   Put the herbs into a blender or food processor and add the salt, lemon juice, preserved lemon rind and flaxseed oil, then process to combine.

5   Add the pine nuts, cucumber, tomatoes and spring onions/scallions to the cauliflower. Pour over the herb dressing and toss well to coat. Scatter over the chopped herbs and serve.

Gut Benefits

The fibre in cauliflower acts as a prebiotic, meaning it provides food for beneficial gut bacteria. Cauliflower contains various antioxidants, including vitamins C and K, and compounds such as glucosinolates and isothiocyanates. These antioxidants help protect the gut lining from oxidative stress and inflammation.

NUTRITIONAL INFORMATION PER SERVING Kcals 619l, **Protein** 23g, **Carbs** 55g of which sugar 23g, **Fat** 31g of which saturates 4.6g, **Fibre** 12g

Harissa Roasted Tofu Salad

Serves: 2

Preparation time: 15 minutes

Cooking time: 40 minutes

2 small sweet potatoes, scrubbed
or peeled and cut into 1cm/½in
chunks (about 400g/14oz)

1 orange pepper, cut into large pieces

1 red pepper, cut into large pieces

1 tbsp olive oil

1 tbsp balsamic vinegar

salt and pepper to taste

8 cherry tomatoes, halved

240g/8½oz firm tofu, cut
into large chunks

Greek or dairy-free yogurt (optional)

HARISSA DRESSING

1 tbsp olive oil

1 tsp harissa paste

1 tbsp lemon juice

a pinch of ground cumin

1 tsp maple syrup

salt and pepper to taste

This dish is delicious hot or cold, so you could prepare it in advance and have it as a packed lunch option. Instead of baking the tofu, you can pan fry or air fry it separately. Tempeh is a great alternative.

1   Preheat the oven to 200°C/400°F/Gas 6.

2   Arrange the sweet potato and peppers in a roasting tray and toss with oil and vinegar. Season with salt and pepper. Roast for 20 minutes.

3   Add the cherry tomatoes and tofu and mix gently. Cook for a further 20 minutes until the tofu turns golden brown.

4   Pour the harissa dressing over the tofu and vegetables. Top with a spoonful of plain yogurt if desired.

5   Serve with mixed salad.

Gut Benefits

Firm tofu is a useful plant protein if you struggle with beans and pulses. The addition of an array of vegetables provides plenty of fibre and prebiotics to support the growth of beneficial gut bacteria.

NUTRITIONAL INFORMATION PER SERVING Kcals 507, Protein 25g, Carbs 42g of which sugars 16g, Fat 24g of which saturates 8.8g, Fibre 12g

Lentil & Goat's Cheese Salad with Roasted Red Peppers

Serves: 2

Preparation time: 15 minutes

2 tbsp cashew nuts

1 x 250g/9oz pouch puy lentils

2 roasted red peppers (from a jar),
    drained and chopped into large chunks

½ red onion, diced

1 handful of parsley, chopped

100g/3½oz mixed salad leaves

1 tbsp roasted chopped
    hazelnuts or walnuts

80g/3oz goat's cheese, crumbled

DRESSING

1 tbsp olive oil

1 tbsp balsamic vinegar

salt and pepper to taste

¼ tsp Dijon mustard (optional)

A quick and easy light salad. Legumes are high FODMAP foods, so are not always suitable for sensitive guts. They are, however, a great source of fibre. You may find a small amount of canned lentils easier to tolerate.

1 Add the lentils, red pepper, onion and parsley to a bowl and mix. Whisk together the dressing ingredients, then pour over the lentil mixture and toss well.

2 Place the mixed leaves on a plate and top with the lentil mixture. Scatter over the cheese and nuts to serve.

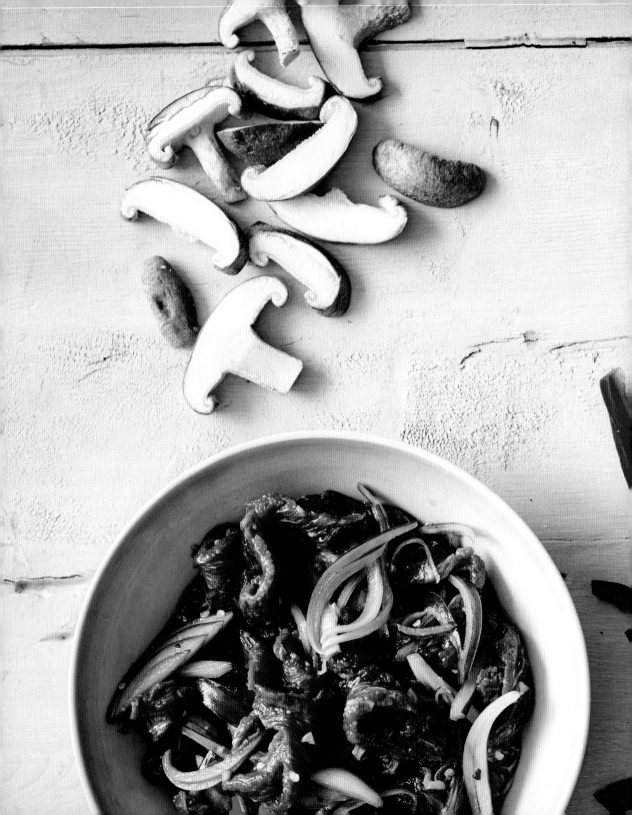

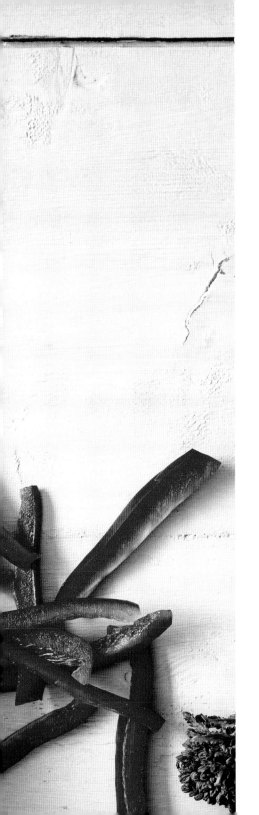

Main Meals

The recipes in this chapter contain a range of family favourites as well as more adventurous creations. Tuck in to my Baked Chicken with Barbecue Sauce or Southern-Spiced Pulled Pork with Sauerkraut. Alternatively, try my Korean Spiced Beef with Kimchi or Vietnamese Prawn & Bacon Fried "Rice". I have also included a number of Paleo vegan options for a lighter choice. You'll love my easy Vegan Mexican Taco Bowl and my Sunflower Seed & Mushroom Falafels with Tahini Lemon Dressing. All are mouth-watering as well as being incredibly nourishing and healing.

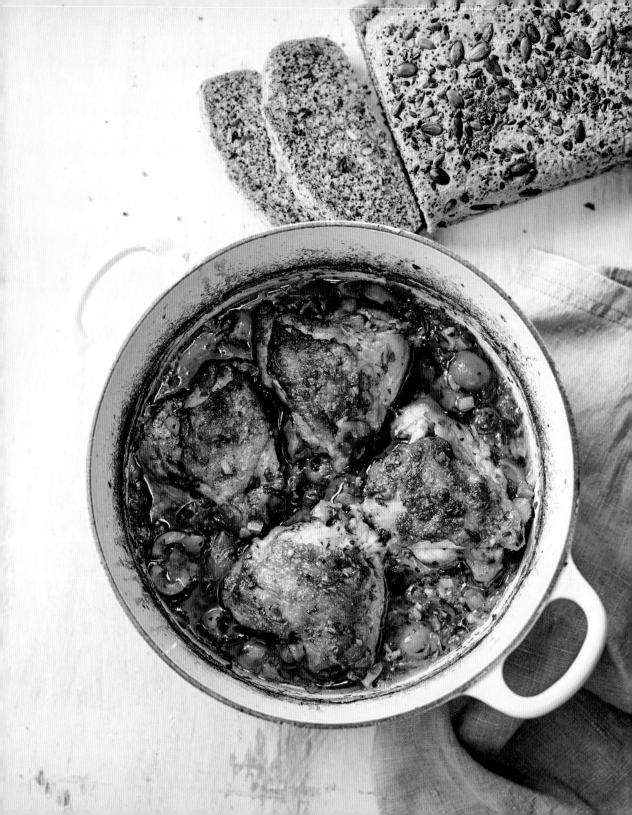

NUTRITIONAL INFORMATION PER SERVING   Kcals 220, Protein 27.7g, Carbs 4.5g of which sugars 3.6g, Fat 10.3g of which saturates 5.3g Fibre 3.3g

Braised Chicken with Green Olives & Preserved Lemon

Serves: 2

Preparation time: 10 minutes

Cooking time: 55 minutes

1 small pinch of saffron threads

4 boneless chicken thighs

1 tbsp olive oil

4 shallots, cut into halves

2 garlic cloves, sliced

¼ tsp ground turmeric

½ tsp ground coriander

½ tsp ground cumin

2 tomatoes, chopped

10 pitted green olives

250ml/9fl oz/1 cup chicken
    bone broth (page 37)

1 preserved lemon, chopped

1 handful of parsley leaves, chopped

sea salt and ground black pepper

Seeded Paleo Bread (page
    66), to serve (optional)

The combination of spices, lemon and herbs provide plenty of flavour for this Turkish-inspired, one-pot dish. It's ideal for a weekday meal because it can be prepared ahead of time. Serve with cauliflower rice (as explained in step 2, page 109) or Paleo bread, if you like. A spoonful of sauerkraut or pickles alongside the dish will give it a probiotic boost.

1   Preheat the oven to 180°C/350°F/Gas 4. Put the saffron in a small mortar and crush using a pestle. Leave to one side.

2   Season the chicken with salt and pepper. Heat the oil in a flameproof casserole over a medium heat and cook the chicken on all sides for 2–3 minutes to brown it. Remove the chicken and leave to one side.

3   Add the shallots, garlic, saffron and spices to the casserole. Cook gently for 5 minutes or until the shallots are soft. Return the chicken to the casserole and scatter over the tomatoes and olives.

4   Pour in the broth and bring to the boil. Cover and cook in the oven for 45 minutes or until the chicken is tender and cooked through. Stir in the preserved lemon and parsley, then serve with Paleo bread, if you like.

Gut Benefits

Olives are a good source of polyphenols to assist the growth of beneficial gut bacteria as well as healthy monounsaturated fats. The dish also contains protein, anti-inflammatory and gut-healing ingredients and healthy fats.

NUTRITIONAL INFORMATION PER SERVING   Kcals 555, Protein 43g, Carbs 17.4g of which sugars 13.8g, Fat 34.5g of which saturates 4g Fibre 12g

Baked Chicken with Barbecue Sauce

Serves: 2

Preparation time: 20 minutes

Cooking time: 50 minutes

100g/3½oz/⅔ cup unblanched almonds

½ tsp smoked paprika

1 tsp garlic powder

olive oil or melted butter, for
    greasing and drizzling

1 egg, beaten

4 skinless, boneless chicken thighs

sea salt and ground black pepper

BARBECUE SAUCE

1 shallot, chopped

1 garlic clove, crushed

200g/7oz/scant ¾ cup canned
    chopped tomatoes

4 tbsp tomato purée/paste

1 eating apple, cored and chopped

60ml/2fl oz/¼ cup balsamic vinegar

1 tsp Dijon mustard

1 tbsp tamari soy sauce or coconut aminos

5mm/¼in piece of root ginger,
    peeled and chopped

½ tsp smoked paprika

Crispy baked chicken tastes great served with a tangy sauce – and it is equally as good served cold for a packed lunch. Serve with a salad. Instead of almonds you can use gluten-free dried breadcrumbs.

1   Preheat the oven to 190°C/375°F/Gas 5. Put all the sauce ingredients into a blender or food processor and blend until reduced to a fine, liquid purée.

2   Transfer the purée to a saucepan over a medium heat and bring to the boil. Reduce the heat, then cover and simmer for 50 minutes, stirring occasionally, until the sauce is thick and darker in colour. (If you like, you can cool the sauce at this point and store it in the fridge for up to 1 week.)

3   Put the almonds into a high-speed blender or food processor and process until fine. Transfer to a shallow bowl and add the paprika and garlic powder, then season with salt and pepper.

4   While the sauce is cooking, line a baking sheet with kitchen foil and put a grill/broiling rack on top. Grease the rack generously with olive oil to prevent the chicken from sticking.

5   Put the beaten egg in a separate shallow bowl. Dip the chicken into the egg, and then coat it thoroughly in the nut mixture.

6   Put the chicken pieces on the rack and drizzle over a little oil. Bake the chicken for 40 minutes or until golden, crisp and cooked through. Serve with the sauce.

Gut Benefits

Tomatoes are rich in antioxidants and vitamin C, and have anti-inflammatory properties. Chicken contains protein and amino acids for gut repair, and selenium for immune regulation.

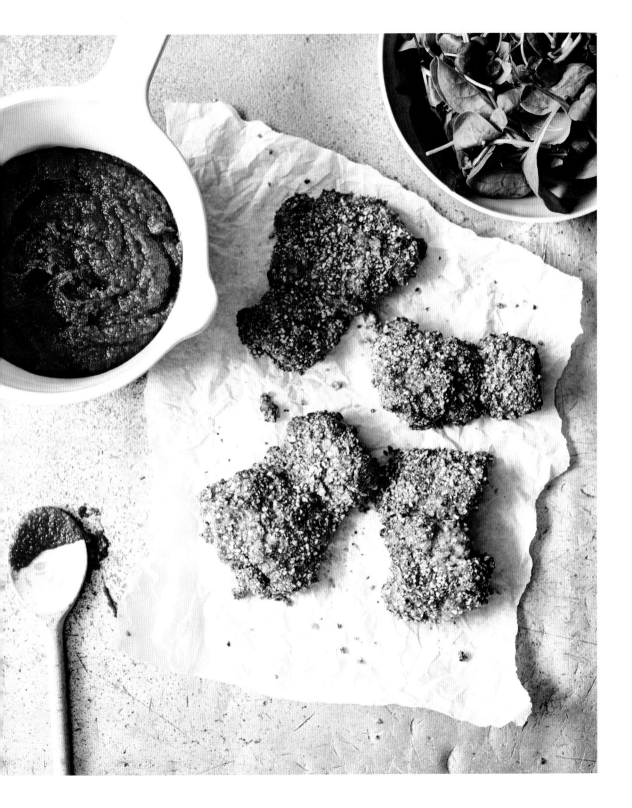

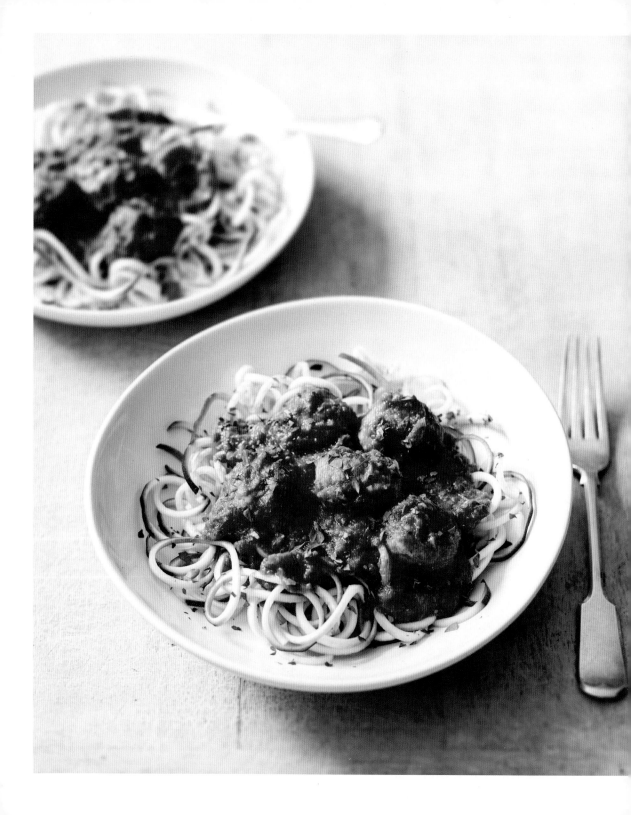

NUTRITIONAL INFORMATION PER SERVING   Kcals 282, Protein 34.5g, Carbs 11.5g of which sugars 10.9g, Fat 10.8g of which saturates 5.4g Fibre 3.6g

Turkey Meatballs with Roasted Tomato Chipotle Sauce

Serves: 2

Preparation time: 20 minutes

Cooking time: 50 minutes

1 small red onion, cut into quarters

2 garlic cloves, peeled and left whole

½ red pepper/bell pepper, deseeded
    and cut into large chunks

500g/1lb 2oz plum tomatoes,
    cut into quarters

2 tsp olive oil or coconut oil

1 tsp chipotle sauce or a few drops
    of Tabasco sauce, to taste

1 tsp lime juice

250g/9oz minced/ground turkey

½ egg, beaten

1 tbsp olive oil

sea salt and ground black pepper

chopped parsley leaves, to serve

This flavourful dish of Italian-style meatballs has a subtle spicy kick from the sauce. You can prepare the sauce and form the meatballs in advance, then reheat the sauce and cook the meat when ready to eat. If you like, serve it with the courgette/zucchini noodles described on page 87 and cooked in water. You could also accompany with pasta or spaghetti if you like.

1   Preheat the oven to 190°C/375°F/Gas 5. Put the onion in a roasting pan and add the garlic, red pepper/bell pepper and tomatoes. Season with salt and pepper, then add the olive oil. Toss the vegetables in the oil to coat, then roast for 30 minutes or until tender and lightly golden.

2   Put the roasted vegetables into a blender or food processor and add the chipotle sauce and lime juice. Blend until smooth, then transfer to a saucepan over a medium-high heat and bring to the boil. Reduce the heat and simmer for 5 minutes. Leave to one side.

3   Put the turkey in a bowl and season with salt and pepper. Add the egg and stir well. Shape into little balls. Heat the coconut oil in a frying pan over a medium-high heat. Fry the balls for 5–6 minutes until browned on all sides. Drain on paper towels.

4   Return the sauce to a gentle simmer, then put the meatballs in the sauce and cook for a further 5 minutes until cooked through. Scatter with parsley and serve.

Gut Benefits

Turkey is a high-protein, low-fat meat that is rich in gut-supporting nutrients, including iron and zinc. It is easy to digest and contains essential amino acids for gut repair.

NUTRITIONAL INFORMATION PER SERVING   Kcals 542, Protein 33.5g, Carbs 14.9g of which sugars 13.9g, Fat 38.4g of which saturates 7.8g Fibre 6.9g

Mandarin Salad of Duck with Green Beans

Serves: 2

Preparation time: 15 minutes, plus
1 hour or overnight marinating

Cooking time: 25 minutes, plus
10 minutes resting

2 duck breasts

2 tsp olive oil

200g/7oz shiitake mushrooms,
   thinly sliced (omit for F)

1 shallot, chopped (omit for F)

1 garlic clove, crushed (omit for F)

2 tbsp balsamic vinegar

2 tbsp olive oil

200g/7oz fine green beans

2 mandarins or 1 orange

2 large handfuls of rocket/
   arugula and watercress

50g/1¾oz/heaped ⅓ cup pine nuts

sea salt and ground black pepper

FIVE-SPICE MARINADE

2 tbsp tamari soy sauce or
   coconut aminos

1 tsp maple syrup or honey

½ tsp ground cinnamon

½ tsp Chinese five-spice powder

Tender duck breasts are cooked with a subtle sauce of Chinese spices. For low FODMAP diets, remove the shallot, garlic and mushrooms (marked as "omit for F"), and replace them with 1 handful of cherry tomatoes, cut into halves; also, use maple syrup instead of honey. Serve the duck with homemade sauerkraut, if you like.

1   Put the marinade ingredients in a shallow dish and combine. Cut a criss-cross pattern into the duck skin and put in the dish. Turn to coat, then leave in the fridge for 1 hour or overnight.

2   Preheat the oven to 200°C/400°F/Gas 6. Heat an ovenproof frying pan over a high heat and add the duck, fat-side down. Brown the skin, then reduce the heat to low and melt the fat for 5 minutes. Transfer to the oven for 10 minutes or until cooked through. Rest the duck on a warm plate for 10 minutes.

3   Meanwhile, heat the coconut oil in a large pan over a medium-high heat. Add the mushrooms and salt and pepper. Cook for 2–3 minutes until caramelized. Add the shallot and garlic, and cook for 3 minutes or until golden. Add the vinegar and oil. Simmer for 5 minutes.

4   Steam the beans in a steamer for 3 minutes or until just tender. Peel the mandarins, or use a sharp knife to remove the skin and pith from the orange. Cut the fruit into thin slices. Slice the duck and serve with the rocket/arugula, watercress, beans and mandarin slices topped with the sauce and pine nuts.

Gut Benefits

Duck contains a number of key vitamins and minerals, including vitamin A, niacin, iron and protein to support a healthy gut.

NUTRITIONAL INFORMATION PER SERVING   Kcals 376, Protein 35g, Carbs 1.3g of which sugars 1.3g, Fat 25.2g of which saturates 4.9g Fibre 0.6g

Southern-Spiced Pulled Pork with Sauerkraut

Serves: 6

Preparation time: 15 minutes

Cooking time: 3½ hours, plus
   30 minutes resting

1.5kg/3lb 5oz pork shoulder on the bone

1 tbsp olive oil, for greasing

1 tbsp sea salt

1 tbsp smoked paprika

1 tsp wholegrain mustard

100ml/3½fl oz/generous ⅓ cup
   apple cider vinegar

1 tsp maple syrup or honey

Little Gem/Bibb lettuce

6 tbsp sauerkraut (page 52), to serve

BALSAMIC DRESSING

1 garlic clove, crushed (omit for F)

100ml/3½fl oz/generous ⅓ cup olive oil

2 tbsp red wine vinegar

1 tbsp balsamic vinegar

1 tsp wholegrain mustard

sea salt and ground black pepper

Slow-cooking the pork makes this dish easy to digest, whether hot or cold. To make this low FODMAP, omit the garlic (marked as "omit for F") and use maple syrup. Instead of sauerkraut, serve with steamed green beans and a leafy salad.

1   Preheat the oven to 220°C/425°F/Gas 7. Score the pork skin about 1cm/½in deep using a sharp knife. Line a roasting pan with a sheet of foil large enough to fold over the pork, then put the pork in the pan. Put the oil in a small bowl and add the salt, paprika and mustard. Mix well, then rub the mixture into the pork. Roast for 20 minutes.

2   Reduce the oven temperature to 160°C/315°F/Gas 2½. Put the vinegar in a bowl and stir in the honey. Pour this mixture over the pork. Re-cover with the foil and return to the oven. Roast for 3 hours or until you can pull the pork apart easily using two forks. Remove the foil and pour off any juices into a bowl.

3   Increase the oven temperature back to 220°C/425°F/Gas 7. Cook the pork, uncovered, for 10 minutes to crisp up the skin. Remove the pork from the oven, cover with foil and leave to rest for 30 minutes. Cut up the crackling and pull the meat apart using forks, discarding any bones or fat.

4   Skim off the fat from the reserved meat juices, then add the dressing ingredients to the bowl and whisk to combine. Drizzle over the pork. Serve the pork on the lettuce and top with a spoonful of the sauerkraut and the crackling.

Gut Benefits

Pork is a good source of digestion-supporting zinc. Using sauerkraut as an accompaniment to dishes is an easy way to increase your intake of fermented foods.

NUTRITIONAL INFORMATION PER SERVING   Kcals 245, Protein 35g, Carbs 6g of which sugars 5.5g, Fat 9g of which saturates 4.9g Fibre 5.9g

Pan-Seared Venison with Blueberries & Broccoli Mash

Serves: 2

Preparation time: 15 minutes

Cooking time: 18 minutes, plus

5 minutes resting

½ tsp thyme leaves, chopped

2 dried juniper berries

a drizzle of olive oil

2 venison steaks, about
    130g/4½oz each, trimmed

2 tsp coconut oil, olive oil
    or ghee (page 38)

½ garlic clove, crushed

100ml/3½fl oz/generous ⅓ cup chicken
    or beef bone broth (page 37)

100g/3½oz/⅔ cup blueberries

sea salt and ground black pepper

BROCCOLI MASH

1 broccoli head, cut into florets

1 tbsp coconut yogurt or
    yogurt (pages 47, 46)

1 tsp finely chopped thyme

1 tbsp chopped parsley

a pinch of garlic powder

Venison is a rich-tasting meat that pairs beautifully with sweet berries. You could use blackberries instead of blueberries when they are in season.

1   Crush the thyme and juniper berries using a mortar and pestle, or bash them on a chopping board using a rolling pin. Transfer to a small dish and stir in a little olive oil. Rub this mixture all over the venison steaks, then season with salt and pepper.

2   Heat the coconut oil in a frying pan over a medium-high heat and cook the venison for 5 minutes. Turn it over and cook for 3–5 minutes more, depending on how rare you like it. Transfer to a warm plate to rest for 5 minutes.

3   Meanwhile, to make the mash, put the broccoli in a steamer and steam over a high heat for 5 minutes or until just tender. Put the broccoli into a blender or food processor and add the yogurt, herbs and garlic powder, then blend to form a mash. Season with salt and pepper and transfer to a pan. Keep warm over a low heat.

4   Add the garlic to the pan for the venison and add the broth and blueberries, then simmer gently for 3 minutes or until the blueberries soften. Slice the venison and serve with the sauce and broccoli mash.

Gut Benefits

Protein-rich venison provides a valuable source of easily absorbable iron and energizing B vitamins. Berries are a good source of polyphenols known to support the growth of beneficial gut bacteria.

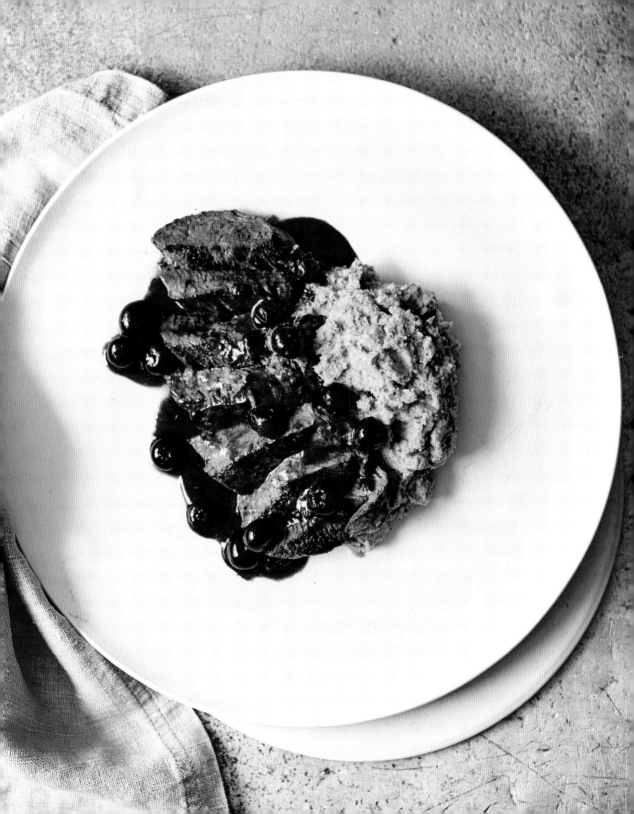

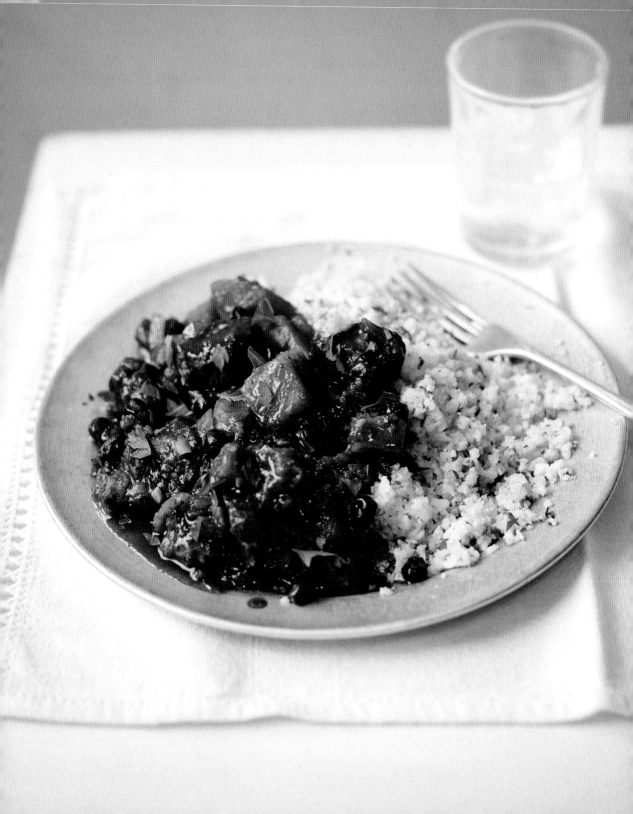

NUTRITIONAL INFORMATION PER SERVING   Kcals 465, **Protein** 35g, **Carbs** 18.7g of which sugars 14.2g, **Fat** 30.6g of which saturates 17.5g **Fibre** 8.2g

Pomegranate Lamb Tagine with Cauliflower Rice

Serves: 2

Preparation time: 20 minutes

Cooking time: 1¾ hours

1 tsp plus 1 tbsp olive oil

300g/10½oz leg of lamb, diced

1 red onion, chopped

1 garlic clove, crushed

5mm/¼in piece of root ginger,
   peeled and grated

1 tsp ground cumin

1 tsp ras el hanout

100g/3½oz butternut squash,
   cut into cubes

250ml/9fl oz/1 cup lamb or beef
   bone broth (page 37)

200g/7oz/scant ¾ cup canned
   chopped tomatoes

60g/2¼oz/⅓ cup dried ready-to-eat
   apricots (optional), chopped

1 tbsp pomegranate molasses

2 tbsp chopped parsley leaves

1 tbsp pomegranate seeds

½ cauliflower, roughly chopped

2 tbsp chicken or beef bone
   broth (page 37)

sea salt and ground black pepper

This Moroccan-style lamb dish is deliciously sweet thanks to the pomegranate, and slow cooking makes it succulent. You can prepare it ahead of time and reheat it when needed. You can also replace the cauliflower rice with basmati rice or quinoa if you like.

1   Heat 1 teaspoon of the oil in a flameproof casserole over a medium-high heat, then add the meat and sear it on all sides for 2–3 minutes. Remove from the pan and leave it on a plate. Add the onion, garlic and ginger to the casserole, and cook for 5 minutes, then stir in the cumin, ras el hanout and squash.

2   Return the meat to the pan and add the broth and tomatoes. Bring to the boil, then add the apricots, if using, and the molasses. Cover and simmer for 1½ hours or until the meat is very tender. Sprinkle with 1 tablespoon of the parsley and the pomegranate seeds.

3   Put the cauliflower into a food processor or electric chopper and process into small rice-like pieces. Heat the 1 tablespoon oil in a frying pan over a medium-high heat. Add the cauliflower and cook for a few seconds to coat it in the oil. Add a splash of broth. Cover and cook for 5 minutes, then uncover, season and simmer, uncovered, for 2 minutes, stirring, until just cooked. Stir in the remaining parsley and serve with the lamb.

Gut Benefits

Slow-cooked dishes are excellent for gut healing. The meat is tender and easy to digest, and the bone broth contains valuable amino acids to support gut health. Add a range of vegetables to the pot to provide antioxidants and soluble fibre.

NUTRITIONAL INFORMATION PER SERVING   Kcals 280, Protein 33.5g, Carbs 15.1g of which sugars 12.2g, Fat 9.5g of which saturates 4.2g Fibre 5.1g

Korean Spiced Beef with Kimchi

Serves: 2

Preparation time: 15 minutes, plus
   30 minutes freezing and 1–2 hours
   marinating

Cooking time: 5 minutes

250–300g/9–10½oz rib-eye
   or sirloin steak

½ red onion, cut in half and sliced

1 tsp olive oil

100g/3½oz purple-sprouting broccoli

½ red pepper/bell pepper,
   deseeded and thinly sliced

2 shiitake mushrooms, sliced

4 handfuls of baby spinach leaves

6 tbsp kimchi (page 54)

KOREAN MARINADE

4 tsp tamari soy sauce or coconut aminos

½ tsp Korean chilli flakes or dried
   chilli/hot pepper flakes

1 tbsp coconut sugar or sugar

2 tsp mirin or rice vinegar

1 tsp sesame oil

1 garlic clove, finely chopped

5mm/¼in piece of root ginger,
   peeled and grated

sea salt and ground black pepper

Kimchi is a spicy fermented food and is good for repopulating the gut as well as being the perfect partner for this traditionally flavoured beef dish. The spinach and broccoli provide cleansing mineral-rich greens, and you could also serve the dish with cauliflower rice (as explained in step 2, page 109).

1   Put all the ingredients for the marinade into a small bowl and stir well to combine. Pour into a shallow dish.

2   Put the steak in the freezer for 30 minutes – it will firm up and be much easier to slice. Slice it thinly, then put it into the marinade with the onion. Marinate in the fridge for 1–2 hours.

3   Heat the coconut oil in a large, heavy frying pan over a medium heat. Add the broccoli and red pepper/bell pepper, and cook for 1–2 minutes until just beginning to soften. Add the mushrooms, beef, onion and the marinade, and stir-fry for 2–3 minutes until the beef is cooked through. Turn off the heat and stir in the spinach leaves. Serve with a spoonful of the kimchi.

Gut Benefits

Including plenty of alkalizing vegetables in your diet, such as spinach, provides valuable phytonutrients, vitamins and minerals to promote gut health and digestive function as well as adding soluble fibre. Shiitake mushrooms are rich in polysaccharides, which help to modulate the immune system and lower inflammation, and vitamin D, which is valuable for gut healing.

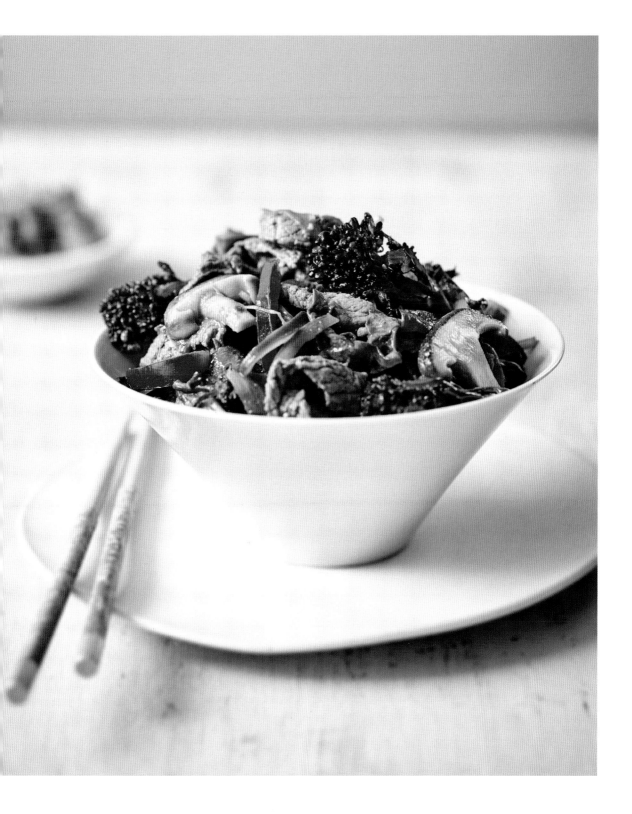

NUTRITIONAL INFORMATION PER SERVING WITH 1 TABLESPOON MAYO   Kcals 471, Protein 26.3g, Carbs 0.8g of which sugars 0.6g, Fat 40.3g of which saturates 18.1g Fibre 0.9g

Beef & Liver Burgers with Wasabi Mayo

Serves: 2

Preparation time: 20 minutes, plus
   30 minutes chilling

Cooking time: 12 minutes

50g/1¾oz chicken livers

200g/7oz minced/ground beef

½ shallot, finely chopped

½ tsp cayenne pepper

½ tsp onion salt

2 tsp Worcestershire sauce

a few drops of Tabasco sauce

1 egg yolk

coconut oil, for shallow-frying

lettuce leaves and tomato slices, to serve

WASABI MAYO

1 egg yolk

¼ tsp Dijon mustard

2 tsp lemon juice

60ml/2fl oz/¼ cup extra virgin
   olive oil or flaxseed oil

50g/1¾oz/¼ cup coconut oil, melted

1–2 tsp wasabi paste or freshly
   grated horseradish, to taste

sea salt and ground black pepper

Liver is highly nutritious and a fabulous healing food for the gut, but it's not always a favourite. Here is a super way to sneak it into your diet. Try to select liver from organic, grass-fed animals. The burgers taste good with homemade pickled dill cucumbers.

1   Trim off any fatty parts and sinew from the chicken livers, then put them into a blender or food processor and process to cut them up finely. Add the beef and season with pepper, then add the shallot and remaining ingredients. Pulse to combine. Using wet hands, shape the mixture into 4 burgers and leave them in the fridge to chill for 30 minutes.

2   To make the mayo, put the egg into a blender or food processor or use a stick blender and beaker. Add the mustard, a pinch of salt, pepper and the lemon juice. Blend together. Combine the oils in a small bowl, then slowly add the oils to the egg mixture while blending slowly. Blend to form a thick mayonnaise. Stir in the wasabi to taste. Leave to one side.

3   Heat the coconut oil for shallow-frying in a non-stick frying pan over a medium-high heat and cook the burgers for 5–6 minutes on each side until thoroughly cooked and the juices run clear. Serve the burgers with the lettuce and tomato, and a spoonful of the wasabi mayonnaise.

Gut Benefits

Liver is rich in protein plus vitamin A – an important vitamin for gut mucosal health and healing. Egg yolk is also rich in healthy fat and nutrients needed for gut function and repair. Both wasabi and fresh horseradish stimulate the digestive juices.

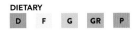
NUTRITIONAL INFORMATION PER SERVING   Kcals 326, Protein 31.6g, Carbs 11.2g of which sugars 11g, Fat 16.5g of which saturates 2.9g Fibre 0.8g

Roasted Whole Salmon with Sweet Soy & Star Anise

Serves: 4

Preparation time: 15 minutes, plus
2 hours marinating

Cooking time: 35 minutes

1 whole salmon, about 1kg/2lb 4oz, cleaned and scaled with head on

110ml/3¾fl oz/scant ½ cup tamari soy sauce or coconut aminos

110ml/3¾fl oz/scant ½ cup rice wine vinegar

4 garlic cloves, crushed (omit for F)

3 spring onions/scallions (green parts only for low FODMAP), finely chopped

3cm/1¼in piece of root ginger, peeled and grated

2 tbsp maple syrup or honey

2 star anise

2 tbsp chopped coriander/cilantro leaves

lime wedges, to serve

A whole salmon is a stunning dish to prepare for a special meal, and this distinctively flavoured version can be served hot or cold. Make this low FODMAP by using maple syrup, only the green tops of the spring onions and omitting the garlic (marked as "omit for F"). Serve with homemade mayonnaise.

1   Wash the salmon under cold running water. Make several diagonal slashes on either side of the fish, then put it in a large dish. Put the remaining ingredients, except the coriander/cilantro, in a bowl and mix well together. Coat the salmon with this marinade, then cover and chill for 2 hours.

2   Preheat the oven to 200°C/400°F/Gas 6. Transfer the salmon to a large piece of foil (large enough to enclose the fish loosely) and spoon over some of the marinade. Loosely cover the fish with the foil to make a parcel, allowing space in the parcel for air to circulate around the fish. Put on a baking sheet and cook in the oven for 30 minutes or until the salmon is cooked through. Preheat the grill/broiler.

3   Open the foil parcel and grill/broil the fish for 2–3 minutes to crisp up the skin. Put the remaining marinade in a small pan over a medium heat and simmer until syrupy. Strain the marinade through a sieve and drizzle over the salmon. Sprinkle with the coriander/cilantro and serve with the lime wedges.

Gut Benefits

Omega-3-rich fish, such as salmon, provides essential fats to maintain the health of the epithelial cells in the digestive tract. These fats (DHA and EPA) also promote healthy gut flora.

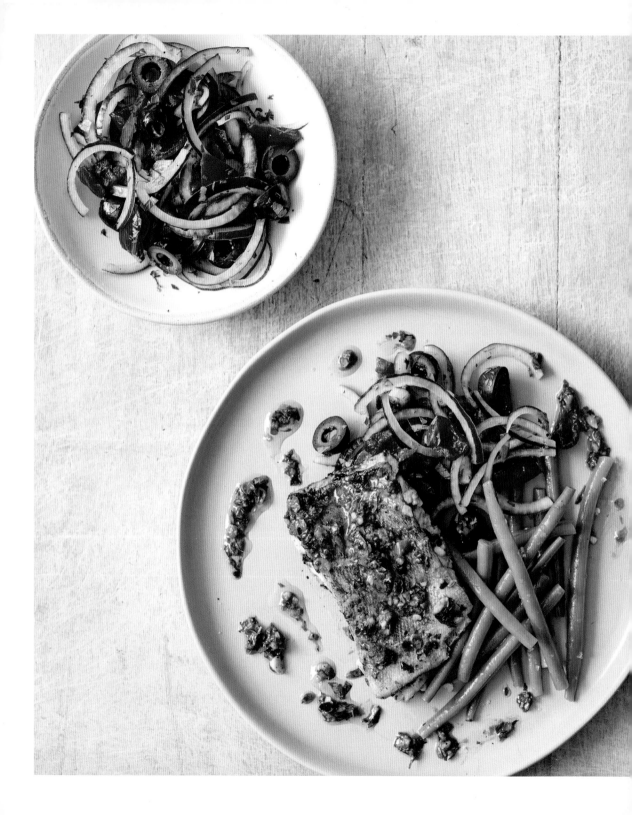

NUTRITIONAL INFORMATION PER SERVING   Kcals 274, Protein 23.3g, Carbs 4.2g of which sugars 3.8g, Fat 17.9g of which saturates 3.9g Fibre 2g

Cod with Mediterranean Herb Dressing

Serves: 2

Preparation time: 15 minutes, plus
   30 minutes marinating

Cooking time: 7 minutes

2 boneless cod fillets, about
   120g/4¼oz each, with skin

½ red onion, cut in half and
   thinly sliced (omit for F)

1 tbsp chopped parsley leaves

1 roasted red pepper/bell pepper
   from a jar, cut into chunks

30g/1oz/¼ cup pitted black
   olives, cut into halves

1 tsp olive oil

sea salt and ground black pepper

HERB DRESSING

1 tbsp capers

1 small anchovy

1 garlic clove (omit for F)

a pinch of dried chilli/hot pepper flakes

1 tbsp mint leaves

1 tbsp coriander/cilantro leaves

1 tbsp parsley leaves

a pinch of stevia or sugar

1½ tbsp balsamic vinegar

3 tbsp extra virgin olive oil

A fresh, herby dressing brings out the delicate flavour of cod, which is served with a simple roasted pepper and onion salad. Make this low FODMAP by omitting the garlic and onion (marked as "omit for F"). Serve with green beans.

1   To make the dressing, put all the ingredients into a blender or food processor. Season with salt and pepper to taste, then blend to combine.

2   Put the fish in a shallow dish and pour over half the dressing. Leave in the fridge to marinate for 30 minutes.

3   To make the salad, put the remaining ingredients, except the oil, in a small bowl and mix well. Leave to one side.

4   Preheat the grill/broiler. Heat the oil in an ovenproof frying pan over a medium heat. Add a little salt and pepper to the pan, then lay in the fish, skin-side up. Cook for 3 minutes, then remove from the heat. Grill/broil for 4 minutes or until the skin blisters and the fish is cooked through. Serve the cod with the salad and the remaining dressing drizzled over.

Gut Benefits

Cod is a source of easy-to-digest protein and, perhaps surprisingly as it is not an oily fish, it also contains omega-3 fats. Vitamin D and selenium, a trace mineral that helps to protect cells from damage, are also present in cod.

NUTRITIONAL INFORMATION PER SERVING   Kcals 408, **Protein** 35.6g, **Carbs** 21.4g of which sugars 16.4g, **Fat** 20.2g of which saturates 4.5g **Fibre** 12g

Cumin-Spiced Halibut with Kale Salad

Serves: 2

Preparation time: 15 minutes

Cooking time: 8 minutes

200g/7oz kale, central stalk
    removed, chopped

1 ripe avocado, pitted and peeled

¼ tsp each garlic powder, cumin
    powder and onion powder

1 tsp coconut syrup, honey
    or maple syrup

1 tbsp tamari soy sauce

2 tbsp lemon juice

1 tbsp nutritional yeast flakes

100g/3½oz/heaped ⅔ cup cherry
    tomatoes, cut into halves

30g/1oz/¼ cup pitted black olives, sliced

30g/1oz/⅓ cup goji berries

30g/1oz/¼ cup toasted sesame seeds

1 tsp olive oil

1 tsp ground cumin

2 halibut steaks

1 tsp olive oil, ghee (page 38) or butter

a pinch of tapioca flour

sea salt and ground black pepper

I adore kale salads – they are so fresh, nourishing and cleansing. This recipe is creamy and lightly spiced, and it makes a wonderful accompaniment to the halibut. You can serve the kale salad on its own as a light snack or side salad.

1   Put the kale in a large bowl and sprinkle over ½ teaspoon salt. Massage the salt into the kale until it wilts. Put the avocado, flavouring powders, syrup, tamari, lemon juice and yeast flakes into a blender or food processor and process to form a thick paste, or put in a bowl and mash together with a fork. Add a dash of water to help it blend, if needed. Spoon it over the kale and use your hands to massage the sauce all over the kale. Toss in the tomatoes, olives, goji berries and seeds.

2   Rub the olive oil and cumin over the halibut steaks and season with salt and pepper. Heat the coconut oil in a large frying pan over a medium-high heat. Dust the fish on both sides with the tapioca flour. Put the fish into the pan, reduce the heat slightly and fry for 4 minutes. Turn the fish over and fry for another 3–4 minutes or until cooked through and crisp. Serve with the kale salad. The salad will keep in the fridge for up to 2 days.

Gut Benefits

Highly nutritious kale is packed with antioxidants and glucosinolates, which protect the gut and support detoxification. Halibut contains protein to nourish the gut and anti-inflammatory omega-3 fats.

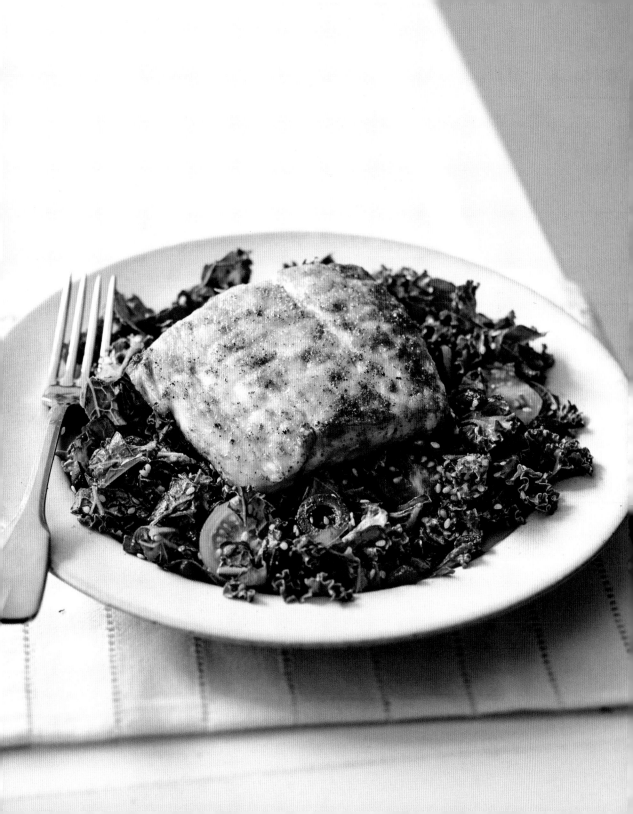

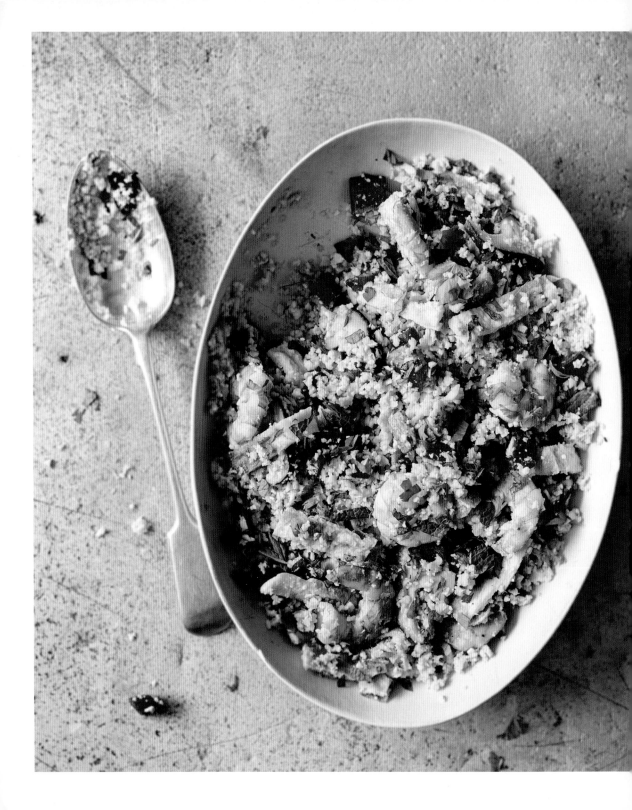

DIETARY

| **D** | **G** | **GR** | **P** |

NUTRITIONAL INFORMATION PER SERVING   Kcals 254, Protein 29.6g, Carbs 7.8g of which sugars 6.5g, Fat 11.5g of which saturates 5g Fibre 5g

Vietnamese Prawn & Bacon Fried "Rice"

Serves: 2

Preparation time: 20 minutes

Cooking time: 15 minutes

½ small cauliflower

200g/7oz shelled raw king
   prawns/jumbo shrimp

2 rashers of unsmoked bacon

2 tsp olive oil

2 eggs, beaten

4 shiitake mushrooms, sliced

½ red pepper/bell pepper,
   deseeded and diced

chopped coriander/cilantro, basil
   and mint leaves, to serve

GINGER AND CHILLI DRESSING

1 garlic clove

1 red chilli, deseeded

5mm/¼in piece of root ginger,
   peeled and grated

1 tsp fish sauce

1 tsp rice wine vinegar

1 tbsp tamari soy sauce or coconut aminos

2 tbsp lime juice

1 tsp coconut sugar, or xylitol,
   stevia or honey

This is a healthy Paleo version of a popular rice dish. Ideally, keep processed meats, such as bacon, to a minimum and use uncured or nitrate/nitrite-free bacon.

1   Put the cauliflower into a food processor and process into small rice-like pieces, then transfer to a large bowl. Put the dressing ingredients into a blender or food processor and blend together. Pour this mixture over the cauliflower in the bowl and mix well.

2   Remove the vein from each prawn/shrimp. Heat a frying pan over a medium-high heat and add the bacon and prawns/shrimp. Cook for 3–4 minutes until the bacon is crispy and the prawns/shrimp are pink and cooked through. Transfer to a plate and keep warm.

3   Heat the coconut oil in the pan and pour in the eggs. Cook for 2–3 minutes, then flip the omelette over and cook briefly on the other side. Remove from the pan. Put on a chopping board and slice thinly. Add to the warmed plate.

4   Add the mushrooms and red pepper/bell pepper to the pan, then the cauliflower with its dressing. Put on the lid and steam-fry for 5 minutes or until the cauliflower is just cooked. Toss in the prawns/shrimp, bacon and egg, and scatter over the herbs to serve.

Gut Benefits

This grain-free, low-allergen dish contains anti-inflammatory spices. The citrus-based dressing will help to stimulate digestive secretions while the prawns/shrimp and eggs ensure that this is a high-protein, nutrient-rich dish.

NUTRITIONAL INFORMATION PER SERVING   Kcals 342, **Protein** 7.8g, **Carbs** 8.2g of which sugars 7.4g, **Fat** 30.8g of which saturates 4.1g **Fibre** 6.5g

Vegan Mexican Taco Bowl

Serves: 2

Preparation time: 15 minutes, plus
   1 hour soaking

Cooking time: 15 minutes

60g/2¼oz/²⁄₃ cup walnuts

2 sun-dried tomatoes, chopped

1 tsp onion powder

½ tsp garlic salt

1 tsp smoked chilli powder

½ tsp ground cumin

½ ripe avocado, peeled

1 cos or romaine lettuce, shredded

1 handful of rocket/arugula

1 celery stalk, thinly sliced

vegan nut cream (savoury version),
   vegan mayonnaise or raw herb cashew
   cheese (pages 48, 39, 49), to serve

ROASTED TOMATO SALSA

1 garlic clove, chopped

½ red onion, chopped

½ green chilli, deseeded and chopped

200g/7oz plum tomatoes,
   cut into quarters

1 tsp olive oil

1 tsp lime juice

sea salt and ground black pepper

A flavoursome taco-style walnut meat goes well with a fresh-tasting roasted salsa and topped with vegan cream, mayo or herb cheese. You can replace the walnut crumble with crumbled cooked tempeh or simply swap for chunks of pan-fried tofu. Serve with Chia, Flaxseed & Tomato Crackers (see page 167) to complete the meal.

1   Soak the walnuts in cold water for 1 hour, then drain and set aside. Preheat the grill/broiler. To make the salsa, put the garlic in a roasting pan and add the onion, chilli and tomatoes. Drizzle with the olive oil and season with salt and pepper. Grill/broil for 10–15 minutes until golden. Put in a blender or food processor and pulse to create a chunky salsa. Stir in the lime juice.

2   Put the walnuts into a high-speed blender or food processor and add the tomatoes, onion powder, garlic salt, chilli powder and cumin. Pulse until combined, but leaving the walnuts in chunky pieces.

3   Cut the avocado into small chunks. Put the lettuce and rocket/arugula in two bowls and top with the celery and avocado. Add the salsa and walnut taco meat. Drizzle over the savoury nut cream and serve.

Gut Benefits

The avocado and nut cream in this dish provide plenty of healthy anti-inflammatory fats, protein and zinc to support gut healing. To help repopulate the gut, choose the nut cheese or add a spoonful of yogurt for the topping instead.

NUTRITIONAL INFORMATION PER SERVING   Kcals 653, Protein 19.2g, Carbs 16.7g of which sugars 7g, Fat 56.7g of which saturates 8.3g Fibre 11g

Sunflower Seed & Mushroom Falafels with Tahini Lemon Dressing

Serves: 2

Preparation time: 20 minutes, plus
   30 minutes chilling

Cooking time: 15 minutes

60g/2¼oz/heaped ⅓ cup macadamia nuts

2 tbsp nutritional yeast flakes

70g/2½oz portobello mushrooms,
   chopped

60g/2¼oz/½ cup sunflower seeds

3 pitted soft dried dates, chopped

2 sun-dried tomatoes in oil, drained

1 tbsp each apple cider vinegar and
   tamari soy sauce or coconut aminos

1 tsp ground cumin

1 handful of parsley leaves

1 garlic clove

30g/1oz/¼ cup sesame seeds

sea salt and ground black pepper

lettuce leaves, to serve

TAHINI LEMON DRESSING

1 tbsp tahini

1 tsp olive oil

1 tsp maple syrup or coconut syrup

1 tbsp lemon juice

These falafels are served with a vegan cheese, rather like Parmesan, and make a healthy low-carb meal packed with healthy fats and nutrients to keep your body energized. Serve them hot or cold – they make an easy packed-lunch option, too.

1   Put the dressing ingredients in a small bowl, add ½ teaspoon black pepper and 1 tablespoon water. Whisk to combine. Leave to one side. Grate the macadamia nuts into a bowl using a fine grater or a Microplane, then stir in half the yeast flakes and ½ teaspoon salt. Leave this vegan Parmesan to one side.

2   Put the mushrooms and seeds into a high-speed blender or food processor and pulse to chop finely. Add ½ teaspoon salt and the remaining yeast flakes and other ingredients, except the sesame seeds, and process to form a soft dough. Wrap in cling film/plastic wrap and chill in the fridge for 30 minutes.

3   Preheat the oven to 180°C/350°F/Gas 4 and cover a baking sheet with baking parchment. Take walnut-size pieces of the mushroom mixture and roll them into balls, then roll the balls in the sesame seeds. Put them on to the prepared baking sheet and transfer to the oven for 15 minutes or until dried out slightly (or pan-fry them in a little oil for 2–3 minutes). Serve the falafels in the lettuce leaves, topped with the dressing and scattered with the vegan Parmesan.

Gut Benefits

Including more plant-based meals is a great way to eat more antioxidant- and fibre-rich vegetables. Mushrooms are a useful vegan source of protein containing gut-supportive vitamin D.

NUTRITIONAL INFORMATION PER SLICE   Kcals 288, Protein 10g, Carbs 10.1g of which sugars 3.8g, Fat 23.1g of which saturates 7.8g Fibre 4g

Spinach, Tomato & Red Pepper Almond-Crusted Quiche

Makes: 1 tart, 6 slices

Preparation time: 20 minutes, plus

   30 minutes chilling

Cooking time: 1 hour, plus cooling

60g/2¼oz/heaped ¼ cup coconut oil or
   butter, diced, plus extra for greasing

125g/4½oz/1¼ cups almond flour

40g/1½oz/⅓ cup tapioca flour

a pinch of salt

a pinch of smoked paprika

1 egg

FILLING

12 cherry tomatoes, cut into halves

a little olive oil, for drizzling

1 tsp coconut oil

150g/5½oz baby spinach leaves

1 tsp chives, chopped

2 roasted red peppers/bell peppers
   from a jar, chopped

1–2 tbsp coconut milk (page 41)
   or coconut cream

4 eggs, beaten

sea salt and ground black pepper

1   Grease a 20cm/8in loose-bottomed tart pan. Put the almond flour into a food processor and add the tapioca, salt and paprika. Season with pepper. Add the coconut oil and process to form breadcrumbs. (Alternatively, rub the coconut oil into the almonds in a bowl by hand or using a pastry cutter, to resemble breadcrumbs.) Add the egg and pulse, or stir, to form a sticky dough. Wrap in cling film/plastic wrap and chill in the fridge for 30 minutes.

2   Preheat the oven to 180°C/350°F/Gas 4. Press the dough into the base and side of the prepared pan. Put baking parchment and baking beans on top. Bake blind for 15 minutes. Remove the beans and bake for 5 minutes or until lightly brown.

3   Meanwhile, make the filling. Put the tomatoes in a roasting pan and drizzle with olive oil. Roast for 15 minutes.

4   Heat the coconut oil in a frying pan over a medium heat. Add the spinach, chives and peppers, and cook briefly until the spinach has wilted. Drain off any liquid.

5   Add the milk to the bowl containing the eggs, and season with salt and pepper. Mix well. Scatter the spinach filling over the base of the flan, then pour over the egg mixture. Arrange the tomatoes cut-side up over the top of the flan. Bake for 40 minutes or until set. Leave to cool slightly before slicing. Serve warm or cold.

Gut Benefits

Vitamin A is essential for the maintenance of the mucosal lining of the intestines, and it supports the innate immune response. Egg yolks and some dairy are good vegetarian sources of vitamin A.

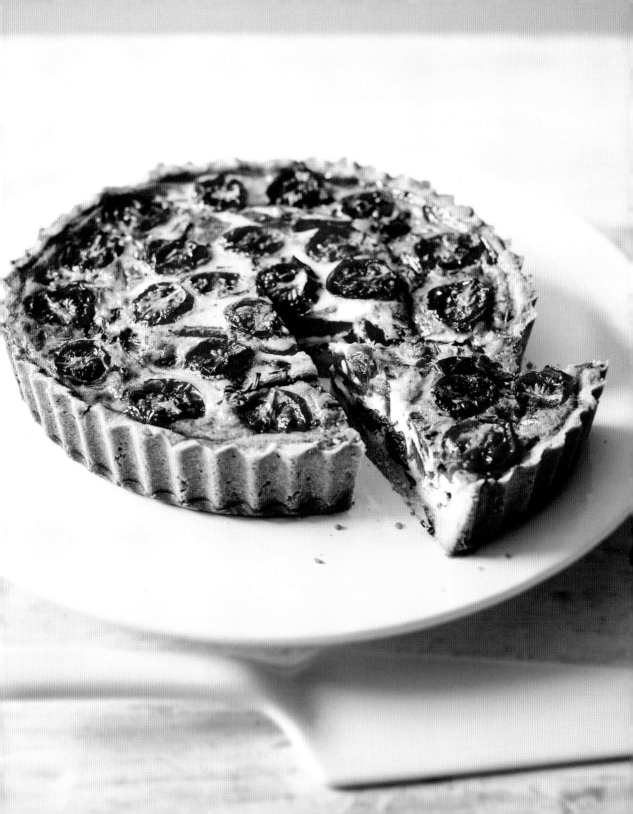

NUTRITIONAL INFORMATION PER SERVING Kcals 519, **Protein** 30g, **Carbs** 69g of which sugars 20g, **Fat** 10g of which saturates 1.8g, **Fibre** 13g

Tempeh & Mushroom Bolognese

Serves: 4

Preparation time: 15 minutes

Cooking time: 55 minutes

This delicious vegan Bolognese is rich in fibre and easy-to-digest plant proteins thanks to the addition of tempeh. You could use tofu or vegan mince if you prefer.

10g/⅓oz dried mushrooms

300g/10½oz tempeh

2 tsp tamari soy sauce

1 tbsp nutritional yeast flakes

2 tbsp olive oil

1 onion, finely diced

2 garlic cloves, crushed

2 short celery stalks, finely diced

3 small carrots, finely diced

350g/12oz chestnut
    mushrooms, finely diced

1 tsp smoked paprika

a pinch of chilli powder or flakes

1 tsp salt

240ml/8fl oz vegetable stock

2 x 400g/14oz cans of chopped tomatoes

black pepper, to taste

TO SERVE

250g spaghetti (gluten free if needed)

1   Cover the dried mushrooms with boiling water and set aside for 10 minutes. Drain, and reserve the liquid. Finely chop the mushrooms.

2   Break up the tempeh and place in a food processor. Pulse very briefly to form chunks. You could also tear it up into small pieces if you prefer. Place in a bowl and drizzle over the soy sauce and nutritional yeast flakes. Toss well.

3   Heat up 1 tbsp olive oil in a large sauté pan. Add the tempeh and cook on a medium heat for 3–4 minutes, stirring occasionally until it browns. Remove from the pan and set aside.

4   Add remaining oil to the pan with the onion and sauté on a low heat for 5 minutes until softened. Add the garlic, celery and carrot, and sauté for another 5 minutes.

5   Add the mushrooms and sauté for a further 5–6 minutes until all of the moisture cooks out and the mushrooms are lightly browned.

6   Add the spices and salt and stir well.

7   Add the mushroom stock and vegetable stock and allow the mixture to bubble for 10 minutes to reduce slightly. Add the tomatoes and allow the mixture to bubble on a medium heat until the tomatoes have reduced by half – about 20 minutes.

8   Add the tempeh and continue to cook for another 5 minutes to reduce the sauce further. Season with black pepper.

9   Meanwhile cook the spaghetti according to instructions and drain.

10 Serve with cooked spaghetti or pasta of choice (gluten free if needed).

Gut Benefits

Tempeh is a fermented soybean product that many people find easier to digest.

NUTRITIONAL INFORMATION PER SERVING Kcals 594, **Protein** 25g, **Carbs** 64g of which sugars 14g, **Fat** 24g of which saturates 3.7g, **Fibre** 8g

Tofu Rice Bowl with Miso-Lemon Dressing

Serves: 2

Preparation time: 15 minutes

Cooking time: 20 minutes

100g/3½oz basmati rice, rinsed

250g/9oz firm tofu, cut into chunks

2 tsp tamari soy sauce

2 tsp nutritional yeast flakes

1 tbsp olive oil

8 shitake mushrooms, sliced

2 baby pak choi/bok choy, halved

4 radishes, finely sliced

1 carrot, grated

2 tbsp pickled sushi ginger slices
   or homemade pickle

1 tbsp chopped toasted peanuts (optional)

1 toasted nori sheet crumbled (optional)

MISO DRESSING

2 tbsp white miso paste

1 tbsp rice wine vinegar

1 tbsp lemon juice

2 tsp olive oil

1 tsp sesame oil

1–2 tsp maple syrup, to taste

½ tsp grated ginger

1 tbsp tamari soy sauce

a little water to thin

This colourful plant-based bowl makes a perfect throw-together meal, and it is a great source of both fibre and probiotics. It is delicious hot or cold, so you can make up a batch and have some for lunch the next day. If you have an air fryer, you can fry the tofu for 3–4 minutes until golden.

1   Place the rice in a pan with about 250ml/8½fl oz water. Bring to the boil, cover, then simmer over a very low heat for 20 minutes. Switch off the heat and allow the rice to steam with the lid on.

2   Make up the dressing by whisking all the ingredients together. Set aside.

3   Place the tofu in a bowl and toss with the tamari soy sauce and nutritional yeast flakes. If using an air fryer, place the tofu chunks in the air fryer for around 4–5 minutes until golden but not too crispy. Alternatively, heat the oil in a non-stick pan and pan fry the tofu, in batches if needed, for about 5 minutes, tossing so that they are golden all over. Remove from the pan.

4   Add the mushrooms to the pan and cook for 3–4 minutes until softened and lightly browned.

5   Steam or blanch the pak choi for 2–3 minutes until just tender.

6   To assemble, divide the rice between two bowls. Top with the tofu and vegetables, then sprinkle over the peanuts and crumbled nori sheet. Drizzle with the dressing to serve.

Gut Benefits

Miso is a traditional Japanese seasoning, fermented with beneficial bacteria such as *Lactobacillus* species and *Aspergillus oryzae*. These probiotics support a healthy gut microbiome, improving digestion and enhancing immune function.

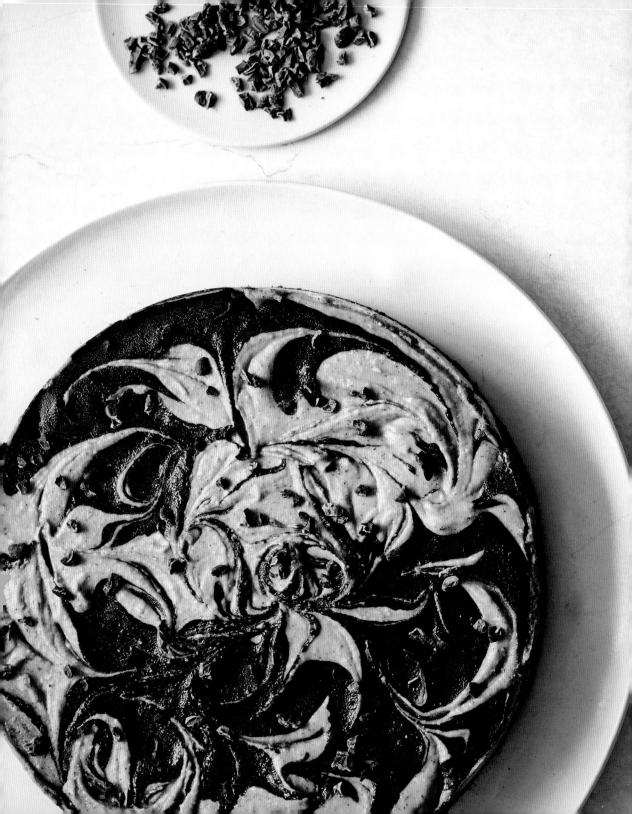

Desserts, Treats & Snacks

Don't feel deprived during the gut-healing programme. Instead, enjoy these fabulous desserts and treats while you nourish and heal your gut. In this chapter you will discover a wealth of delicious, mouth-watering sweet dishes and healthy snacks. Try my light and refreshing Mint & Chocolate Ice, cut yourself a slice of the Raw Mango, Turmeric & Cardamom Tart, munch on homemade Chocolate Bounty Bites or Fruity Gummy Sweets. For a savoury snack, make a batch of my delicious Barbecue Kale Crisps or homemade crispbreads. All are packed with healing nutrients to support your digestion.

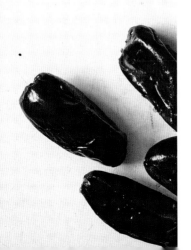

5-STEP

REPL   REPO   REPA   REB

DIETARY

D   G   GR   P   V   VE

NUTRITIONAL INFORMATION PER SERVING   Kcals 134, **Protein** 3.6g, **Carbs** 15.8g of which sugars 6.6g, **Fat** 7.6g of which saturates 1.6g **Fibre** 2.8g

Lemon Balm & Berry Ice

Serves: 4

Preparation time: 10 minutes, plus

  6 hours freezing

60g/2¼oz/½ cup cashew nuts

300ml/10½fl oz/scant 1¼ cups

  coconut kefir or kefir (page 44)

200g/7oz/1²/₃ cups mixed berries

2 tbsp xylitol, caster sugar or maple syrup

zest and juice of 1 lemon

1 handful of lemon balm leaves

Put all the ingredients, except the lemon balm, into a blender or food processor and blend until smooth. Add the lemon balm and pulse. Pour into a freezerproof container and freeze for 2 hours. Whisk, then freeze, and whisk once more. Freeze again. (Alternatively, use an ice cream maker according to the manufacturer's instructions.)

Gut Benefits

Using kefir as the base of this ice cream is an easy way to repopulate the gut with beneficial bacteria. Milk or kefir also provides additional protein and healthy fats.

5-STEP

REM   REPA   REB

DIETARY

D   G   GR   P   V   VE

NUTRITIONAL INFORMATION PER SERVING   Kcals 198, **Protein** 2.7g, **Carbs** 14.7g of which sugars 3.3g, **Fat** 15.8g of which saturates 5.7g **Fibre** 3.1g

Mint & Chocolate Ice

Serves: 4

Preparation time: 10 minutes, plus

  6 hours freezing

2 ripe avocados, pitted and peeled

250ml/9fl oz/1 cup coconut milk

½ tsp peppermint extract

1 tsp matcha green tea powder (optional)

1 handful of mint leaves

2 tbsp xylitol, caster sugar or coconut syrup

50g/1¾oz/¹/₃ cup dairy-free,

  sugar-free chocolate chips

Put all the ingredients, except the chocolate chips, into a blender or food processor and blend until smooth. Stir in the chocolate. Pour into a freezerproof container and freeze for 2 hours. Whisk, then freeze, and whisk once more. Freeze again. (Alternatively, use an ice cream maker according to the manufacturer's instructions.)

Gut Benefits

For additional gut healing, add 30g/1oz/scant ¼ cup glutamine powder.

NUTRITIONAL INFORMATION PER SERVING Kcals 331, **Protein** 6.9g, **Carbs** 32.9g of which sugars 22.4g, **Fat** 19.3g of which saturates 5.8g **Fibre** 6.7g

Granola Fruit Bowl

Serves: 2

Preparation time: 10 minutes, plus
   3 hours or overnight freezing

A crunchy, nutty topping contrasts beautifully with the smooth, fruity layer beneath. You could also serve this antioxidant-rich and super-healthy dessert for breakfast.

1 banana

150g/5½oz/1¼ cups frozen mixed berries

1 tsp maca powder (optional)

½ tsp ground cinnamon

1 tbsp almond nut butter

150ml/5fl oz/scant ⅔ cup coconut kefir,
   kefir or coconut milk (pages 44, 41)

1 Chop the banana and put it into a freezer bag. Exclude all the air, then seal and freeze for 3 hours or overnight until solid.

2 Put the banana into a blender or food processor and add the remaining ingredients. Blend until smooth. Serve topped with the granola, goji berries and coconut flakes.

GOJI GRANOLA TOPPING

1 handful of Pumpkin & Cinnamon
   Paleo Granola (page 68)

1 tbsp goji berries

1 handful of coconut flakes

Gut Benefits

Adding maca powder supports adrenal health while the nut butter provides healthy fat and protein. Bananas are a good source of soluble fibre and a traditional fruit to ease diarrhoea.

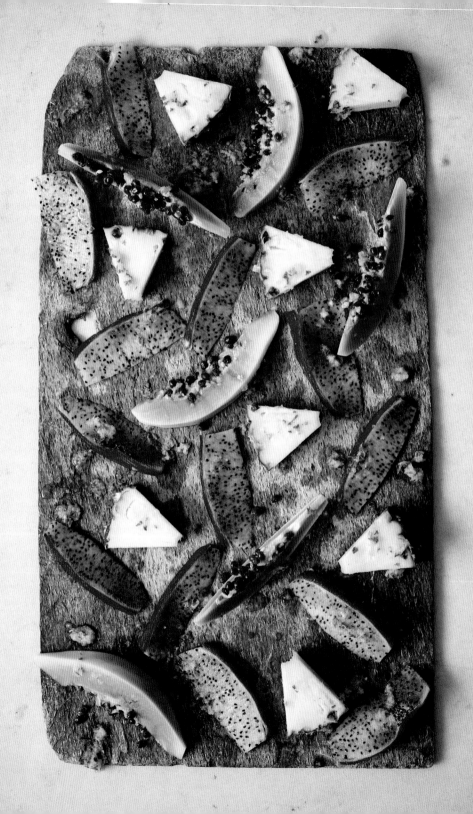

NUTRITIONAL INFORMATION PER SERVING   Kcals 85, **Protein** 1.1g, **Carbs** 26.4g of which sugars 19.5g, **Fat** 0.2g of which saturates 0g **Fibre** 8g

Tropical Fruit Platter with Sweet Ginger & Mint Dressing

Serves: 2

Preparation time: 10 minutes

½ papaya, peeled, seeded and sliced

100g/3½oz pineapple, cut into wedges

1 dragon fruit or 6 lychees,
    peeled and sliced

yogurt, coconut yogurt (pages 46, 47) or
    vegan nut cream (page 48), to serve

GINGER AND MINT DRESSING

2.5cm/1in piece of root ginger,
    peeled and grated

10 mint leaves, finely chopped

grated zest and juice of 1 lemon

1 tbsp coconut syrup or maple syrup

Fresh and simple to prepare, this dish has the piquancy of ginger in the sweet dressing and it contains fruits that are particularly helpful for supporting the digestion.

1   To make the dressing, put all the ingredients in a small bowl and mix together well.

2   Arrange the fruit on a platter and pour over the dressing, then serve with yogurt.

Gut Benefits

Papaya and pineapple both contain digestive enzymes and fibre, which aid bowel health by lowering inflammation and soothing the digestive tract, while the ginger has anti-inflammatory properties. Serving the fruit with homemade yogurt or coconut yogurt gives it an additional probiotic boost.

5-STEP

| REM | REPL | REPO | REPA | REB |

DIETARY

| D | G | GR | P | S |

NUTRITIONAL INFORMATION PER SERVING   Kcals 398, Protein 8.4g, Carbs 42.6g of which sugars 41.7g, Fat 22.4g of which saturates 16.2g Fibre 6.3g

Cherry & Coconut Layered Parfait

Serves: 2

Preparation time: 10 minutes, plus cooling and 1 hour chilling

Cooking time: 5 minutes

150ml/5fl oz/scant ⅔ cup pure pomegranate juice

2 tsp gelatine

200g/7oz/heaped ¾ cup coconut yogurt (page 47)

500g/1lb 2oz/2½ cups pitted frozen cherries

1 tbsp goji berries

1 tbsp coconut flakes

Creamy coconut yogurt pairs beautifully with cherries for this naturally sweet, layered dessert. It's delicious as a breakfast dish, too. Soy yogurt is a good vegan alternative and has a higher protein content. You can use agar-agar flakes instead of gelatine for a vegan option. If you can tolerate dairy, using plain or Greek yogurt is a great choice.

1   Put the pomegranate juice in a small pan over a medium heat and bring to the boil. Reduce the heat to a simmer and whisk in the gelatine. Simmer until the gelatine dissolves completely, whisking constantly. Remove from the heat and leave the mixture to cool to room temperature.

2   Pour into a blender or food processor and add the yogurt and half the cherries. Blend until smooth. Chill in the fridge for 1 hour or until it starts to thicken.

3   Put the remaining cherries in a small pan over a medium heat and cook gently for 1–2 minutes, breaking them up a little with a spoon. Put a little of the coconut mixture into two glasses. Top with a spoonful of the cherry compote and repeat the layers once more. Scatter over the goji berries and coconut flakes, and serve.

Gut Benefits

Cherries are packed with antioxidants to facilitate healing and lower inflammation. The yogurt helps to repopulate the gut with friendly bacteria.

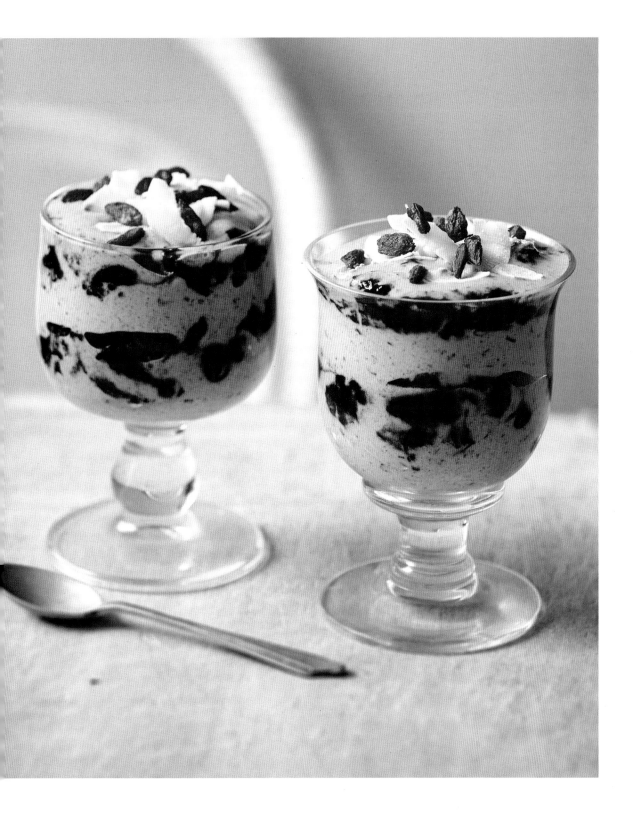

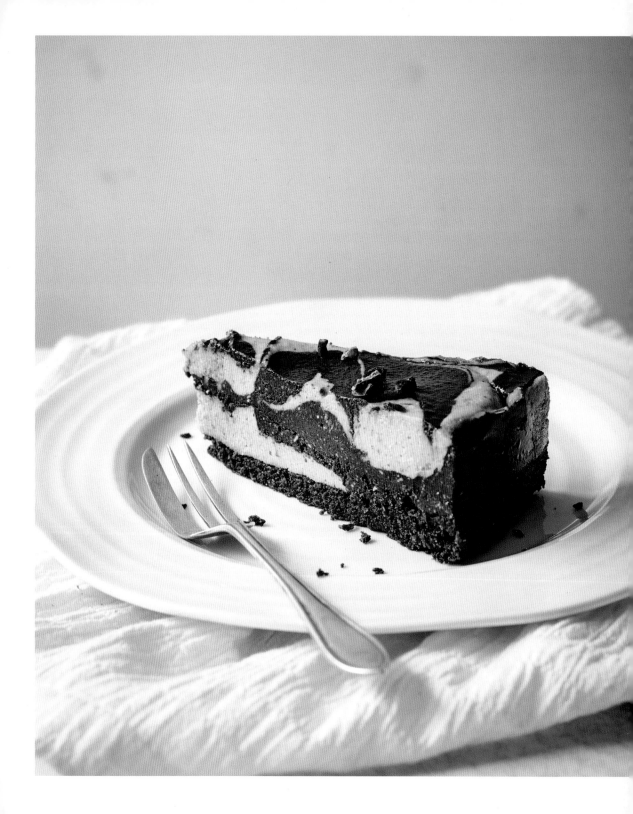

NUTRITIONAL INFORMATION PER SLICE   Kcals 479, Protein 8.8g, Carbs 28.6g of which sugars 16.3g, Fat 37.3g of which saturates 11.6g Fibre 6.6g

Mocha Swirl Cheesecake

Makes: 1 cheesecake, 12 slices
Preparation time: 25 minutes, plus
   2–4 hours soaking, 4–5 hours freezing
   and 1 hour chilling

coconut oil, for greasing
200g/7oz/2 cups pecan nuts
30g/1oz/⅓ cup raw cacao powder
120g/4¼oz/ heaped ⅔ cup pitted
   soft dried dates, chopped
cacao nibs, to decorate

CHEESECAKE LAYERS
300g/10½oz/2⅓ cups cashew nuts
250ml/9fl oz/1 cup coconut milk or
   coconut yogurt (pages 43, 49)
125g/4½oz/heaped ⅔ cup
   pitted soft dried dates
4 tbsp almond nut butter
2 tbsp lucuma powder (optional)
1 tbsp vanilla extract
100g/3½oz/scant ½ cup raw
   cacao butter, melted
30g/1oz/⅓ cup raw cacao powder
1 tbsp dandelion coffee granules
   or instant coffee granules
70g/2½oz/⅓ cup coconut oil, melted
2 tbsp xylitol, caster sugar
   or stevia, to taste

The coffee alternative in this cheesecake, dandelion root, is good for gut health. It supports bile flow and is known for its gentle laxative effect. It is also caffeine-free. Here it is combined with cacao to create an indulgent-tasting dessert.

1   Soak the nuts for the cheesecake layers for 2–4 hours in water, then drain and leave to one side. Lightly grease a 22cm/8½in springform cake pan. Put the pecan nuts into a high-speed blender or food processor and process until fine. Add the cacao powder and dates, and process until the mixture just combines. Add a dash of water if needed.

2   Tip into the base of the prepared pan and press down firmly. Chill in the fridge while you prepare the layers.

3   To make the caramel layer put half the soaked cashew nuts into a blender or food processor and add 150ml/5fl oz/scant ⅔ cup of the coconut milk, the dates, nut butter, lucuma and vanilla. Process until smooth. Add the cacao butter and blend until smooth and creamy. Transfer to a bowl and clean the blender.

4   Put all the remaining ingredients, including the remaining milk and cashews, into the blender and process until smooth to make the mocha layer. Spoon one-third of the caramel mixture in blobs over the crust. Repeat with one-third of the mocha filling.

5   Alternate the layers until the filling is used up. Use a knife to swirl the fillings gently together to make a marbled effect. Put in the freezer for 4–5 hours to firm up, then transfer to the fridge for 1 hour. Scatter over the cacao nibs. Serve in slices.

Gut Benefits
Dandelion root has bile- and liver-supporting properties.

NUTRITIONAL INFORMATION PER SERVING   Kcals 416, Protein 7.3g, Carbs 16.4g of which sugars 15.9g, Fat 35.7g of which saturates 10.7g Fibre 7.5g

Apple & Plum Crisp

Serves: 6

Preparation time: 15 minutes

Cooking time: 50 minutes

8 plums, pitted and sliced

4 eating apples, cored,
    peeled and chopped

1 tbsp lemon juice

2 tsp ground cinnamon

2 tbsp maple syrup, honey
    or coconut syrup

150g/5½oz/1 cup unblanched almonds

a pinch of sea salt

60g/2¼oz/heaped ¼ cup
    coconut oil, melted

100g/3½oz/1 cup pecan nuts, chopped

coconut yogurt or vegan nut cream
    (pages 47, 48), to serve

This crunchy fruit dessert is similar to a crumble but uses nuts instead. You can also use the nut topping for other fruits including berries or frozen fruits when fresh fruits are out of season. Nuts provide plenty of magnesium and zinc, making this great for supporting mood, too.

1   Preheat the oven to 180°C/350°F/Gas 4. Put the plums and apples in a shallow baking dish and add the lemon juice, 1 teaspoon of the cinnamon and 1 tablespoon of the maple syrup. Mix together well.

2   Put the almonds into a high-speed blender or food processor and grind until very fine. Put in a large bowl and add the salt and the remaining cinnamon. Stir to combine. Mix in the oil, remaining maple syrup and the pecans. Scatter the mixture evenly over the fruit. Bake for 40–50 minutes until golden and crisp. Serve with yogurt.

Gut Benefits

Apples are known for their gut-healing properties. Rich in polyphenols and pectin, a type of soluble fibre, they help to lower inflammation and promote the growth of beneficial bacteria in the gut.

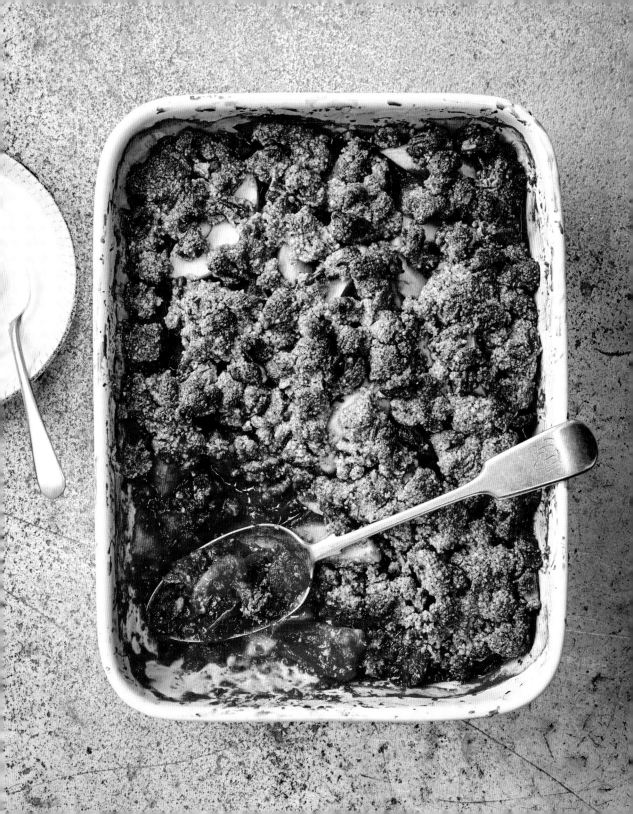

NUTRITIONAL INFORMATION PER SLICE   Kcals 418, **Protein** 8g, **Carbs** 16g of which sugars 11g, **Fat** 36g of which saturates 16.3g **Fibre** 4.5g

Raw Mango, Turmeric & Cardamom Tart

Makes: 1 tart, 12 slices

Preparation time: 20 minutes, plus
   overnight soaking and 4–5 hours
   freezing

300g/10½oz/2⅓ cups cashew nuts

1 tbsp coconut oil, plus extra for greasing

150g/5½oz/1 cup unblanched almonds

125g/4½oz/1 cup raisins

50g/1¾oz/heaped ½ cup desiccated/
   dried shredded coconut

½ tsp ground cardamom

1 tbsp vanilla extract

150g/5½oz/scant ⅔ cup coconut
   cream or coconut yogurt (page 47)

juice of 1 orange, or 70ml/2¼fl oz/
   generous ¼ cup water kefir or
   kombucha (pages 45, 43)

2 ripe mangos, peeled, pitted and
   chopped, plus extra to decorate

100g/3½oz/½ cup coconut oil, melted

70g/2½oz/scant ⅓ cup raw
   cacao butter, melted

½ tsp ground turmeric

Turmeric is a potent anti-inflammatory spice and surprisingly delicious combined with sweet mango and creamy cashew nuts in this sweet and fruity raw tart. You can serve the tart frozen or defrosted as a chilled dessert. Instead of cashew nuts you could use silken tofu.

1   Soak the cashew nuts overnight in water, then drain and leave to one side. Lightly grease a 22cm/8½in springform cake pan. Put the almonds into a high-speed blender or food processor and pulse until roughly chopped. Add the oil and the raisins, coconut, cardamom and vanilla, and process until the mixture starts to come together.

2   Press this crust mixture evenly into the base of the prepared pan, then put it in the fridge to chill while you make the filling.

3   Put the soaked cashews into a blender or food processor and add the coconut cream, orange juice and mangos. Blend together, then add the remaining ingredients and blend until smooth.

4   Pour the mixture onto the crust and smooth the top. Put in the freezer for 4–5 hours to firm up. Transfer to the fridge 1 hour before serving. Remove from the springform pan. Decorate with mango. Store in the fridge and eat within 4 days.

Gut Benefits

The fermented foods provide beneficial bacteria. Turmeric is an excellent anti-inflammatory spice for the gut, and the coconut oil contains healthy fats with antimicrobial properties.

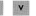
NUTRITIONAL INFORMATION PER SLICE Kcals 275, **Protein** 5.9g, **Carbs** 12.5g of which sugars 6.7g, **Fat** 22.7g of which saturates 5.8g **Fibre** 4.8g

Raw Orange Brownie Slices

Makes: 12 slices

Preparation time: 20 minutes, plus
    2 hours freezing

Cooking time: 2 minutes

coconut oil, for greasing

125g/4½oz/heaped ¾ cup
    unblanched almonds

125g/4½oz/1¼ cups pecan nuts

30g/1oz/scant ⅓ cup raw cacao
    powder or chocolate vegan
    or whey protein powder

100g/3½oz/½ cup pitted soft dried dates

a pinch of sea salt

1 tbsp vanilla extract

zest of 1 orange

100g/3½oz/⅔ cup dairy-free sugar-
    free chocolate chips (optional)

ORANGE TOPPING

130g/4½oz/1 cup cashew
    nuts or silken tofu

juice of 1 small orange

60g/2¼oz/heaped ¼ cup
    coconut oil, melted

3 tbsp maple syrup or a little stevia

These protein-packed slices are ideal as a snack. They are a good source of vitamin C to support adrenal health and act as an antioxidant. If you prefer a stronger orange flavour, add 2 drops of pure orange extract when you prepare the topping.

1 Grease and line a 20cm/8in square cake pan with baking parchment. Put the nuts into a high-speed blender or food processor and pulse until coarsely ground. Add the remaining ingredients, except the chocolate chips, to the blender and process until the mixture forms a dough.

2 Put the mixture into the prepared pan and press down firmly. Put the pan in the freezer while you prepare the topping.

3 Put the topping ingredients into a high-speed blender or food processor and blend until smooth. Pour the mixture over the base. Smooth the top, then put back in the freezer for 1–2 hours to harden.

4 Remove from the freezer and allow to soften slightly before cutting into 12 slices. Melt the chocolate chips, if using, in a heatproof bowl over a pan of gently simmering water, making sure the base of the bowl doesn't touch the bottom of the pan. Drizzle the melted chocolate over the brownies. Serve or store in the fridge for up to 3 days or freeze for up to 3 months.

Gut Benefits

Nuts are a useful source of fibre and prebiotics, as well as antioxidants and magnesium.

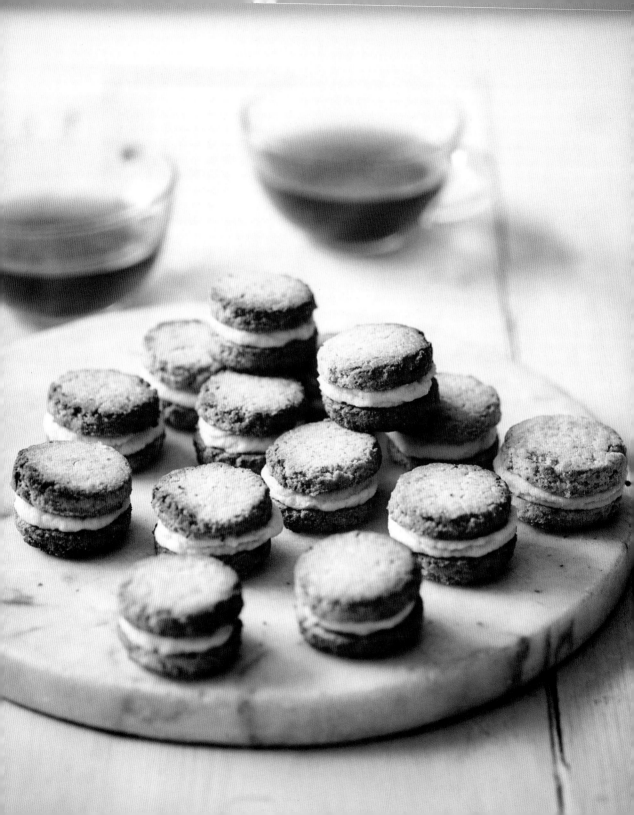

NUTRITIONAL INFORMATION PER COOKIE   Kcals 123, Protein 3.3g, Carbs 10.8g of which sugars 0.8g, Fat 8.1g of which saturates 4.6g Fibre 1.5g

Lemon Cream Sandwich Cookies

Makes: about 14 cookies

Preparation time: 30 minutes

Cooking time: 20 minutes, plus cooling

30g/1oz/¼ cup coconut flour

30g/1oz/scant ¼ cup tapioca flour

30g/1oz/¼ cup arrowroot

30g/1oz/scant ¼ cup vanilla vegan
    or whey protein powder

1 tsp gluten-free baking powder

½ tsp bicarbonate of soda/baking soda

zest and juice of 2 lemons

1 tbsp lucuma powder (optional)

2 tbsp xylitol or caster sugar

1 heaped tbsp chia seeds

60g/2¼oz/heaped ¼ cup
    coconut oil, melted

LEMON FILLING

1 quantity vegan nut cream (page 48)
    using zest and juice of 2 lemons instead
    of water, and sweetener adjusted

These coconut-based cookies are sandwiched with a simple lemon nut cream. They are perfect as a little sweet something after a meal and for lunch boxes.

1   Preheat the oven to 180°C/350°F/Gas 4. Line a baking sheet with baking parchment. Sift the flours, arrowroot, protein powder, baking powder and bicarbonate of soda/baking soda into a large bowl.

2   Add the lemon zest, lucuma, if using, and xylitol, and mix well. Put the chia seeds in a bowl with the lemon juice and soak for 2 minutes. Add the chia mixture to the large bowl followed by the coconut oil, and mix well to form a dough.

3   Roll out the dough between two sheets of baking parchment. Stamp out 28 circles 4cm/1½in in diameter and put them on the prepared baking sheet. Bake for 20 minutes or until lightly golden. Transfer to a wire rack to cool completely.

4   Make up the nut cream as described on page 48 using the lemon zest and juice instead of water, and add sweetening to taste. Spread 14 of the cookies with 1 tablespoon of the filling for each, then put a plain cookie on top. Serve. Store in the fridge for up to 1 week.

Gut Benefits

Adding chia seeds to cookie mixes is a great way to increase the fibre, particularly in grain-free or gluten-free recipes.

NUTRITIONAL INFORMATION PER SLICE   Kcals 454, Protein 10.1g, Carbs 29.9g of which sugars 22.1g, Fat 33.2g of which saturates 18.7g Fibre 6.5g

Paleo Carrot & Ginger Cake

Makes: 1 large cake, 12 slices

Preparation time: 30 minutes, plus
   24 hours chilling

Cooking time: 50 minutes, plus cooling

2 × 400ml/14fl oz cans full-fat
   coconut milk

150g/5½oz/¾ cup coconut oil or
   butter, plus extra for greasing

100g/3½oz/⅔ cup canned
   pineapple, drained

100g/3½oz/½ cup pitted soft dried dates

10 eggs

100g/3½oz/⅓ cup maple syrup or honey

60g/2¼oz/½ cup coconut flour

100g/3½oz/1 cup ground almonds

1 tsp bicarbonate of soda/baking soda

zest of 1 orange

1 tsp ground cinnamon

3 tsp vanilla extract

350g/12oz carrots, finely grated

50g/1¾oz stem ginger, chopped

100g/3½oz/scant 1 cup goji berries

70g/2½oz/¾ cup walnuts, chopped

3 tbsp xylitol

coconut flakes, to decorate

1   Put the cans of coconut upright in the fridge for 24 hours.

2   Preheat the oven to 180°C/350°F/Gas 4. Grease and line two 23cm/9in springform cake pans with baking parchment. Put the pineapple into a blender or food processor with the dates, eggs, coconut oil and maple syrup, and blend until smooth. Add the coconut flour, almonds, bicarbonate of soda/baking soda, orange zest, cinnamon and 2 teaspoons of the vanilla. Blend.

3   Stir in the carrots, ginger, goji berries and walnuts. Pour into the prepared baking pans and bake for 50 minutes or until golden brown and a skewer inserted into the middle comes out clean. Transfer the cakes to a wire rack to cool completely.

4   Take the coconut milk out of the fridge and open the can. Gently scoop out the coconut cream from the top and put it in a bowl. (Use the remaining liquid in smoothies.) Grind up the xylitol in a blender or food processor until very fine.

5   Using a stick blender, whip the coconut cream for 1 minute or until light and fluffy. Whip in the xylitol and remaining vanilla, then put it in the fridge until ready to use. Spread a little of the cream on top of one of the cakes. Put the other cake on top and spread the remaining cream over the top. Toast the coconut flakes for decoration in a pan over a medium heat for 2 minutes or until lightly golden. Sprinkle them over the cake.

Gut Benefits

Carrots contain carotenoids and vitamin A, which support the mucosa in the gut, and antioxidants, which help to lower inflammation. Cooking carrots makes them more digestible and may also make their key nutrients more easily absorbed by the body.

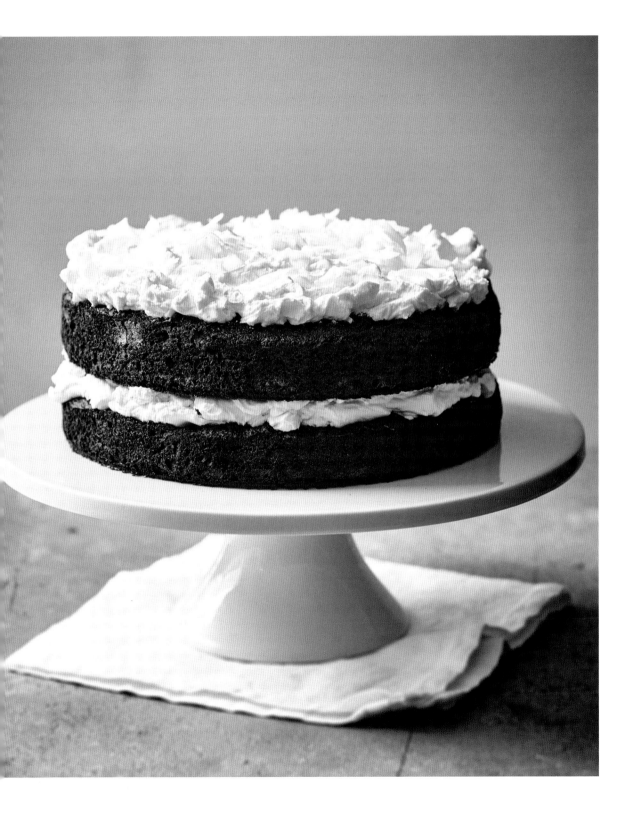

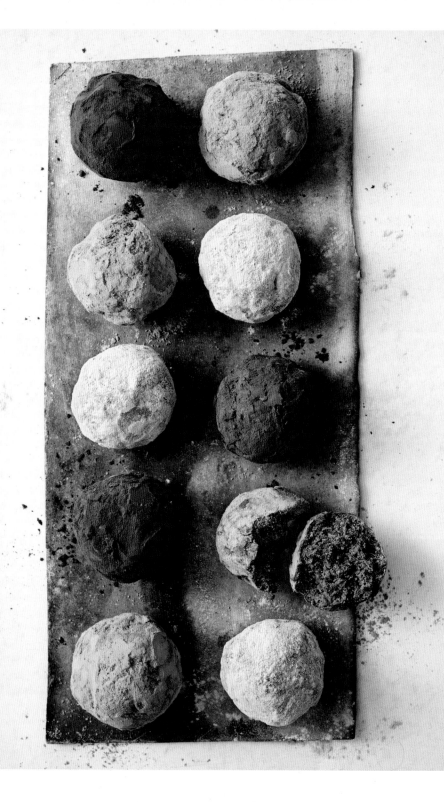

NUTRITIONAL INFORMATION PER BITE   Kcals 161, Protein 5.5g, Carbs 17g of which sugars 5g, Fat 9.7g of which saturates 3g Fibre 1.3g

Matcha Superfood Bites

Makes: 10 bites

Preparation time: 20 minutes, plus
   15 minutes soaking and 30 minutes
   chilling

60g/2¼oz/⅓ cup xylitol or soft
   brown sugar/caster sugar
60g/2¼oz/½ cup dried
   cherries or goji berries
120g/4¼oz/½ cup cashew nut butter
zest of 1 lemon
1 tbsp lemon juice
1 tsp matcha green tea powder
a pinch of sea salt
2 tbsp raw cacao powder, lucuma
   powder or goji berry powder
60g/2¼oz/heaped ¼ cup raw cacao
   butter or coconut oil, melted
30g/1oz/scant ¼ cup plain, vanilla or
   chocolate vegan protein powder,
   colostrum powder or collagen powder
½ tsp vanilla extract
matcha green tea powder, lucuma
   powder or cacao powder, for dusting

These antioxidant-packed nuggets are ideal for lowering inflammation. Matcha has anti-inflammatory effects on the digestive system making it a useful choice for improving gut health. The raw cacao butter makes the snacks rich and creamy – an indulgent healing treat.

1   Line a baking sheet with baking parchment. Put the xylitol into a blender or food processor and grind very finely. Soak the cherries in warm water for 15 minutes. Drain.

2   Put the cashew nut butter into a food processor or a bowl and add the xylitol, lemon zest and juice, matcha, salt, cacao powder and cacao butter. Pulse, or stir, to combine. Add the cherries and the remaining ingredients, and process, or stir, to form a dough. Chill in the freezer for 30 minutes to firm up.

3   Use a spoon to scoop out walnut-size pieces. Roll into balls and put on the prepared baking sheet. Roll the truffles in a little matcha powder or use some or all of the powders for dusting. Serve or store in the fridge for up to 1 week.

Gut Benefits

Nut butters are incredibly nutrient dense. Cashew nut butter contains magnesium, which supports the nervous system, making it ideal for helping with stress. Matcha green tea provides anti-inflammatory catechins and L-theanine to relieve anxiety.

NUTRITIONAL INFORMATION PER BITE   Kcals 242, **Protein** 4.7g, **Carbs** 7.7g of which sugars 3.2g, **Fat** 21.7g of which saturates 16.6g **Fibre** 3.4g

Chocolate Bounty Bites

Makes: 10 bites

Preparation time: 20 minutes, plus
   1½ hours freezing

Cooking time: 3 minutes

150g/5½oz/1²/₃ cups desiccated/
   dried shredded coconut

2 tbsp collagen powder, or vanilla
   or plain vegan protein powder
   or glutamine powder

70g/2½oz/⅓ cup coconut oil

a pinch of sea salt

3 tbsp maple syrup

a pinch of stevia, to taste (optional)

1 tsp vanilla extract

CHOCOLATE COATING

200g/7oz/1¼ cups dairy-free,
   sugar-free chocolate chips

1 tsp coconut oil

Make these tempting sweet treats as a healthy version of a popular chocolate bar. They contain collagen powder, which is a good supplement to support gut healing. They freeze well and defrost quickly, so they make a handy snack to store.

1   Line a baking sheet with baking parchment. Put half the coconut into a high-speed blender or food processor and process until very fine. Add the rest of the coconut and the remaining ingredients to the processor and process to combine – keeping some texture.

2   Shape the mixture into 10 walnut-size balls. Put on the prepared baking sheet and freeze for 1 hour to firm up.

3   Melt the chocolate chips with the coconut oil in a small saucepan over a low heat. Remove the balls from the freezer. Dip each ball into the chocolate and return them to the baking parchment. Return to the freezer for 15 minutes or until the chocolate has set.

4   Repeat the chocolate coating once more and return the balls to the freezer for 10 minutes to set. Serve when the second coat is just set to avoid them becoming too hard. Store the balls in the fridge for up to 1 week or freeze them for up to 3 months.

Gut Benefits

Adding collagen or glutamine powder is a great way to support gut healing and increase your intake of important amino acids. Coconut provides antimicrobial properties and healthy fats to nourish the digestive system.

NUTRITIONAL INFORMATION PER SWEET   Kcals 13, Protein 1.4g, Carbs 1.7g of which sugars 1.6g, Fat 0g of which saturates 0g Fibre 0.5g

Fruity Gummy Sweets

Makes: 20 candies

Preparation time: 10 minutes, plus at least 1 hour chilling

Cooking time: 3 minutes

juice of 1 lemon

200g/7oz/1 cup frozen cherries
   or berries, defrosted

1 tbsp maple syrup, honey
   or stevia, or to taste

30g/1oz/¼ cup gelatine powder

100ml/3½fl oz/generous ⅓ cup water
   kefir or kombucha (pages 45, 43)

These little candies are perfect as a sweet treat. You can use stevia if you prefer to keep the sugar content low. They are ideal as a healthy snack or a sweet treat, and they make a great treat for children.

1   Use silicone moulds or line a 20cm/8in baking sheet with baking parchment. Put the lemon juice and cherries into a blender or food processor and blend until completely mixed.

2   Pour the mixture into a saucepan. Add the maple syrup and gelatine, and whisk together. Gently heat the mixture until the gelatine has dissolved, stirring constantly. Remove from the heat and whisk in the kefir, or use a blender briefly to ensure the mixture is smooth.

3   Pour into the moulds or onto the sheet. Put in the fridge for at least 1 hour to firm up. Remove the gummies from the moulds or, if you used a baking sheet, cut the mixture into bite-size pieces. Serve or store in the fridge for up to 1 week.

Gut Benefits

Using gelatine is a great way to add healing support to these delicious candies. The addition of kefir provides beneficial bacteria, whereas the cherries and berries are packed with anti-inflammatory polyphenols to help support the growth of friendly bacteria.

NUTRITIONAL INFORMATION PER CRISPBREAD   Kcals 122, **Protein** 4.6g, **Carbs** 2.7g of which sugars 0.5g, **Fat** 12.2g of which saturates 3g **Fibre** 3g

Fennel & Poppy-Seed Crispbreads

Makes: 12 crispbreads

Preparation time: 15 minutes

Cooking time: 25 minutes, plus cooling

60g/2¼oz/heaped ⅓ cup
   unblanched almonds

60g/2¼oz/½ cup cashew nuts

1 tbsp coconut flour

30g/1oz/¼ cup pumpkin seeds

30g/1oz/¼ cup sunflower seeds

30g/1oz/¼ cup sesame seeds

2 tbsp poppy seeds

2 tbsp fennel seeds

½ tsp sea salt

2 tbsp coconut oil, melted

1 egg, beaten

Serve these nut-based crispbreads with spreads, homemade mayonnaise, a spoonful of fermented vegetables or to accompany salads and soups. Seeds are a great source of healthy fats and zinc to support gut healing and mood.

1   Preheat the oven to 180°C/350°F/Gas 4 and line a baking sheet with baking parchment. Put the almonds, cashews and coconut flour into a high-speed blender or food processor and grind up finely.

2   Pulse in the seeds and salt until almost fully ground, but leave a little texture. Transfer to a bowl. Add the oil and gradually add the egg to form a soft ball of dough.

3   Roll out the dough between two pieces of baking parchment to 5mm/¼in thick. Cut into rectangular crispbreads about 5cm/2in in length.

4   Bake for 20–25 minutes until golden and crisp. Transfer to a wire rack to cool completely. Serve or store in an airtight container for up to 1 week.

Gut Benefits

These protein-rich crispbreads contain healthy fats as well as healing minerals, including zinc and iron. The fennel seeds can help to alleviate bloating and flatulence.

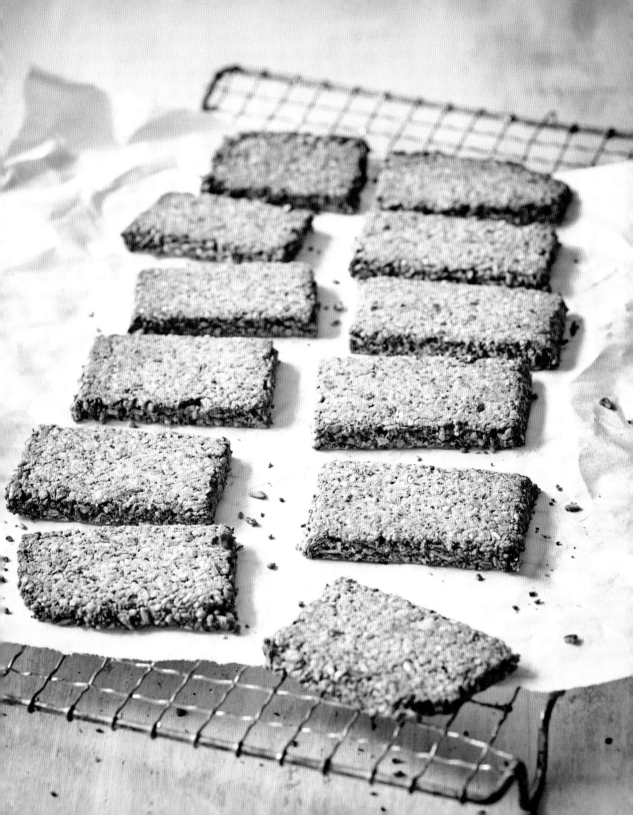

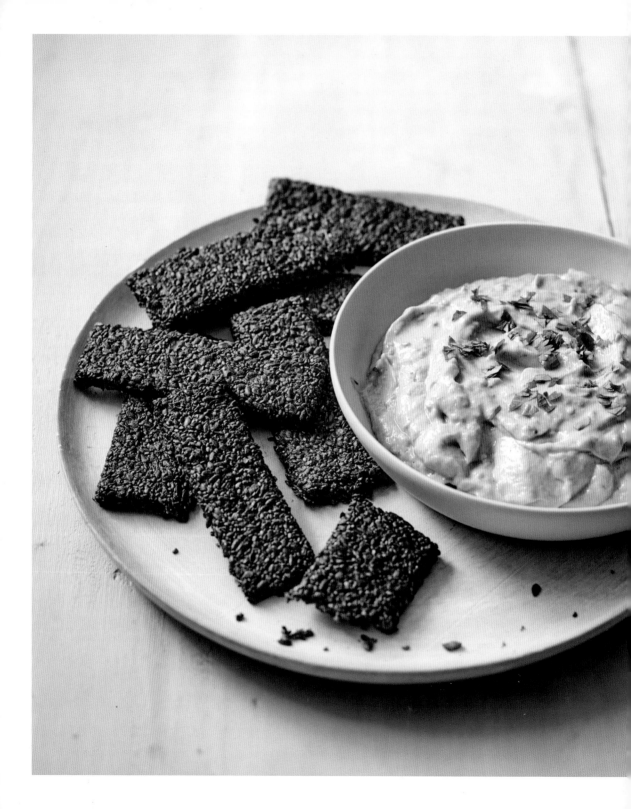

NUTRITIONAL INFORMATION PER CRACKER   Kcals 69, **Protein** 2.3g, **Carbs** 4.1g of which sugars 0.8g, **Fat** 5.1g of which saturates 0.6g **Fibre** 3.4g

Chia, Flaxseed & Tomato Crackers

Makes: 24 crackers

Preparation time: 15 minutes

Cooking time: 45 minutes, plus cooling

50g/1¾oz/scant ½ cup pumpkin seeds

70g/2½oz/½ cup chia seeds

160g/5¾oz/1 cup flaxseed

1 red pepper/bell pepper,
    deseeded and chopped

4 sun-dried tomatoes in oil, drained

2 tomatoes, chopped

3 tbsp lemon juice

1 tsp ground cumin

2 tbsp tamari soy sauce or
    coconut aminos

½ tsp garlic salt

These spicy seeded crackers go well with soups and stews as well as serving as a snack with Chipotle Avocado Cream Spread, homemade mayonnaise, nut butters or nut cheese. They are delicious with a spoonful of fermented vegetables or pickles too.

1   Preheat the oven to 150°C/300°F/Gas 2. Line a baking sheet with baking parchment. Put all the ingredients into a high-speed blender or food processor and add 60ml/2fl oz/¼ cup water. Blend to form a stiff paste.

2   Put the mixture onto the prepared baking sheet, then spread it out to about 5mm/¼in thick using damp hands to make a rectangle shape. Mark the mixture into rectangular cracker shapes using a knife. Bake for 40–45 minutes until crisp. Transfer to a wire rack to cool completely. Serve or store in an airtight container for up to 1 week.

Gut Benefits

These grain-free crackers contain soluble fibre and protein thanks to the addition of the seeds, making them useful for supporting the digestion.

NUTRITIONAL INFORMATION PER SERVING Kcals 141, **Protein** 3.1g, **Carbs** 3.2g of which sugars 2.5g, **Fat** 13.1g of which saturates 4.1g **Fibre** 2.8g

Chipotle Avocado Cream Spread

Serves: 2

Preparation time: 5 minutes

1 chipotle pepper in adobo sauce, drained

1 tomato

1 avocado, cut in half, pitted,
   peeled and roughly chopped

4 tbsp coconut yogurt (page 47)
   or Greek yogurt

¼ tsp ground cumin

1 tbsp chopped coriander/cilantro leaves

sea salt and ground black pepper

Spicy, sweet, creamy and fresh-tasting, this dip tastes good with vegetable sticks or as a topping for baked fish. Also, serve it with Paleo breads or crackers. Avocado is a great source of healthy fats and B vitamins to support mood, too. (Picture on page 166.)

1   Put all the ingredients, except the corriander/cilantro leaves, into a blender or food processor and blend until smooth. Season to taste.

2   Transfer to a serving bowl and sprinkle with the coriander/cilantro, then serve. Store in the fridge for up to 3 days.

Gut Benefits

The healthy monounsaturated fats and vitamin E in avocado help to lower inflammation, and its fibre supports bowel health. You can also add avocado oil to veggies to dramatically improve the absorption of their antioxidants and fat-soluble vitamins across the gut. Using yogurt in the spread is a great way to boost its probiotic content.

5-STEP
REM **REPL** REPA

DIETARY
D G **GR** P S V **VE**

NUTRITIONAL INFORMATION PER SERVING   Kcals 216, Protein 10.8g, Carbs 15.1g of which sugars 9g, Fat 12.3g of which saturates 1.6g Fibre 7.8g

Barbecue Kale Crisps

Serves: 2

Preparation time: 10 minutes, plus
2–4 hours soaking

Cooking time: 25 minutes, plus cooling,
or 10–12 hours dehydrating

30g/1oz/¼ cup sunflower seeds

coconut oil, for greasing

2 tbsp nutritional yeast flakes

4 small pitted soft dried dates

1 tbsp tamari soy sauce or coconut aminos

1 tbsp apple cider vinegar

1 tsp ground cumin

½ tsp onion powder

¼ tsp garlic salt

½ tsp smoked paprika

3 sun-dried tomatoes, drained

¼ red pepper/bell pepper,
deseeded and chopped

1 tbsp lemon juice

100g/3½oz kale, chopped

Homemade kale crisps are nutritious and surprisingly easy to make – and they are much cheaper than shop-bought versions. Here, kale pieces are coated in a creamy, tangy sauce and then baked. If you have a dehydrator, you can dehydrate them overnight until crisp and dry.

1   Soak the sunflower seeds in cold water for 2–4 hours, then drain. Preheat the oven to 150°C/300°F/Gas 2 and grease a baking sheet. Put the sunflower seeds and all the other ingredients, except the kale, into a blender or food processor and blend until smooth.

2   Put the kale in a bowl and pour over the sauce. Thoroughly combine the kale with the sauce until all the kale is coated. Arrange the kale in a single layer on the baking sheet and bake for 15 minutes.

3   Remove from the oven and flip the kale crisps over. Bake for 5–10 minutes more until crisp, watching carefully to make sure that the kale doesn't burn. Remove from the oven and leave on the baking sheet to cool completely. (Alternatively, if you have a dehydrator, spread the kale over teflex sheets in a dehydrator and dry for 10–12 hours.)

Gut Benefits

Kale is packed with nutrients to support gut health, including beta-carotene, flavonoids such as quercetin, vitamins A, K and C, and magnesium. It is a good source of fibre and it provides food for beneficial bacteria and aids detoxification.

NUTRITIONAL INFORMATION PER SERVING   Kcals 56, Protein 1.4g, Carbs 5.3g of which sugars 5g, Fat 3.2g of which saturates 0.4g Fibre 2.8g

Beetroot Cumin Crisps

Serves: 2

Preparation time: 5 minutes, plus
  10 minutes soaking

Cooking time: 20 minutes, plus cooling,
  or 18–22 hours dehydrating

2 beetroots/beets

1 tbsp apple cider vinegar

2 tsp olive oil

1 tsp ground cumin

sea salt and ground black pepper

Creating your own vegetable crisps is simple and makes a popular and delicious snack. You can bake these in the oven, air fry them or dehydrate them if you have a dehydrator. This recipe will work well with other root vegetables, too. Use a mandoline, if possible, to create thin slices.

1   Preheat the oven to 180°C/350°F/Gas 4 and line a baking sheet with baking parchment. Thinly slice the beetroot/beets with a mandoline or a very sharp knife. Put the cider vinegar and olive oil in a bowl and mix together. Toss the beetroot/beet in the vinegar mixture and leave to soak for 10 minutes.

2   Spread the beetroot/beet slices on the prepared baking sheet and season with salt, pepper and cumin. Bake for 15–20 minutes until crispy, turning them over halfway through cooking. Transfer to a wire rack to cool completely. (Alternatively, if you have a dehydrator, spread them out over teflex sheets in a dehydrator and dry for 10–12 hours. Flip them over and dry for a further 8–10 hours until crispy.)

Gut Benefits

Beetroot/beet is incredibly healthy. Loaded with vitamins A, B and C, it is also high in fibre, manganese and folate. It is also a rare source of phytonutrients called betalains, which have been shown to have antioxidant, anti-inflammatory and detoxification qualities. It's ideal for supporting cleansing and bile function, too.

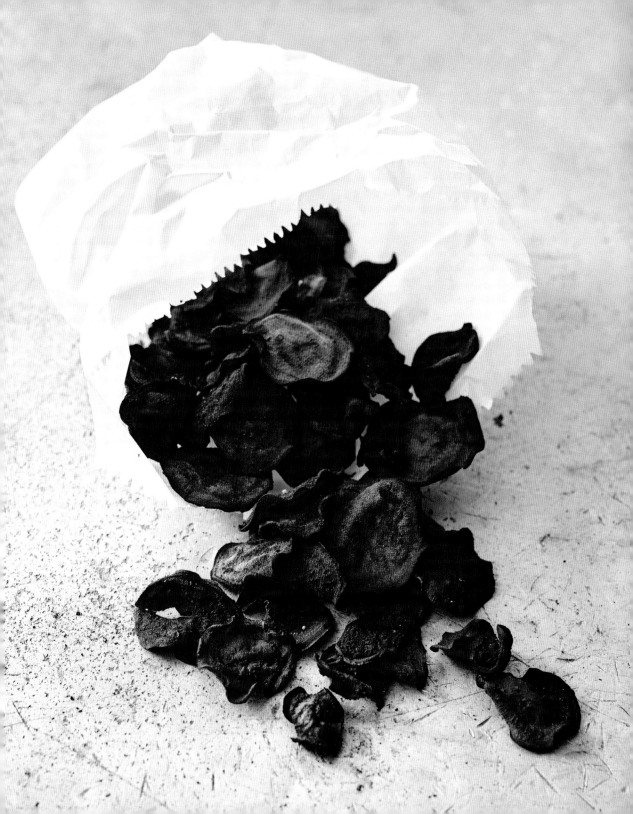

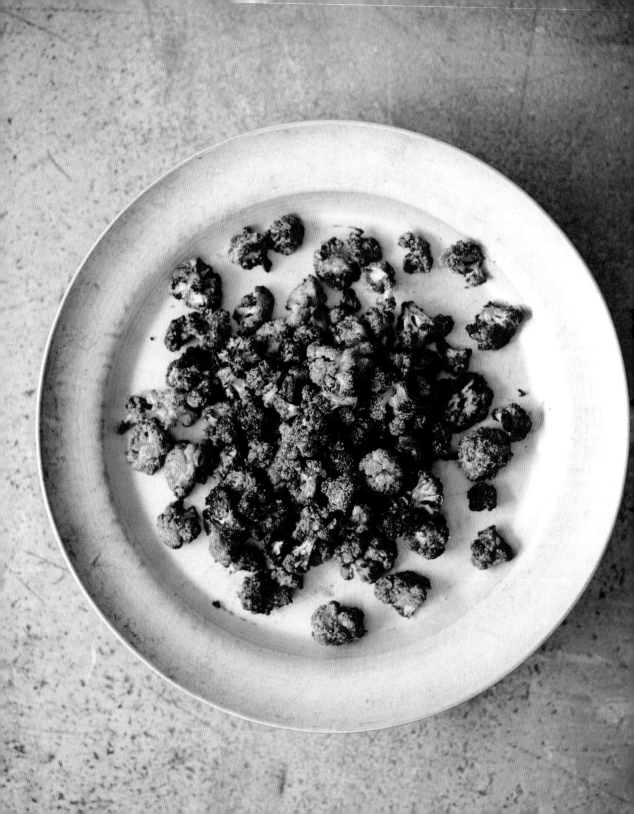

NUTRITIONAL INFORMATION PER SERVING   Kcals 86, Protein 6.6g, Carbs 4.9g of which sugars 4.2g, Fat 4.8g of which saturates 0.8g Fibre 1.4g

Crispy Cauliflower Popcorn

Serves: 6

Preparation time: 10 minutes

Cooking time: 45 minutes, plus cooling

1 small cauliflower

2 tsp extra virgin olive oil, melted butter,
    ghee (page 38) or coconut oil

1–2 tbsp nutritional yeast flakes
    (optional), to taste

½ tsp smoked paprika

½ tsp ground cumin

¼ tsp ground turmeric

½ tsp sea salt

ground black pepper

Cauliflower is tossed in spices and oil, and baked until crisp for these moreish snacks. You could also vary the flavourings: for a sweet version, blend together 4 pitted soft dried dates with 1 tablespoon almond nut butter and ½ teaspoon ground cinnamon, loosened with a little water.

1   Preheat the oven to 180°C/350°F/Gas 4. Line a baking sheet with baking parchment. Break the cauliflower into small popcorn-size pieces.

2   Put the remaining ingredients in a large bowl and season with pepper. Mix together well. Add the cauliflower and mix to coat thoroughly.

3   Spread the cauliflower over the prepared baking sheet and bake for 45 minutes or until golden brown and crispy, turning occasionally. Remove from the oven and leave on the baking sheet to cool completely.

Gut Benefits

Cauliflower and other brassica vegetables, such as broccoli and cabbage, are great for supporting detoxification.

Notes

1 Takakura, W and Pimentel, M, "Small intestinal bacterial overgrowth and irritable bowel syndrome: An update", *Frontiers in Psychiatry*, 11, 2020. doi:10.3389/fpsyt.2020.00549

2 Kim, G, Lee, K and Shim, J O, "Gut bacterial dysbiosis in irritable bowel syndrome: A case-control study and a cross-cohort analysis using publicly available data sets", *Microbiology Spectrum*, 11, 2023

3 Voreades, N, Kozil, A and Weir, T L, "Diet and the development of the human intestinal microbiome", *Frontiers in Microbiology*, 5(494), 2014. doi: 10.3389/fmicb.2014.00494. PMID: 25295033; PMCID: PMC4170138

4 Takakura, W and Pimentel, M, "Small intestinal bacterial overgrowth and irritable bowel syndrome: An update", *Frontiers in Psychiatry*, 11, 2020. doi: 10.3389/fpsyt.2020.00549

5 Pimentel, M et al., "Methane production during lactulose breath test is associated with gastrointestinal disease presentation", *Digestive Diseases and Sciences*, 48(1), 2003, pp.86–92. doi: 10.1023/a:1021738515885. PMID: 12645795

6 Ghoshal, U C, Shukla, R and Ghoshal, U, "Small intestinal bacterial overgrowth and irritable bowel syndrome: A bridge between functional organic dichotomy", *Gut Liver*, 11(2), 2017, pp.196–208. doi: 10.5009/gnl16126. PMID: 28274108; PMCID: PMC5347643

7 Martinez Jason, E et al., "Unhealthy lifestyle and gut dysbiosis: A better understanding of the effects of poor diet and nicotine on the intestinal microbiome", *Frontiers in Endocrinology*, 12, 2021. doi: 10.3389/fendo.2021.667066

8 Zeissig, S et al., "Changes in expression and distribution of claudin 2, 5 and 8 lead to discontinuous tight junctions and barrier dysfunction in active Crohn's disease", *Gut*, 56(1), 2007, pp.61–72. doi: 10.1136/gut.2006.094375. Epub 2006 Jul 5. PMID: 16822808; PMCID: PMC1856677

9 Fasano, A et al., "Zonulin, a newly discovered modulator of intestinal permeability, and its expression in coeliac disease", *Lancet*, 355(9214), 2000, pp.1518–1519. doi: 10.1016/S0140-6736(00)02169-3. PMID: 10801176

10 Fasano, A, "Leaky gut and autoimmune diseases", *Clinical Reviews in Allergy & Immunology*, 42(1), 2012, pp.71–78. doi: 10.1007/s12016-011-8291-x. PMID: 22109896

11 Turcotte, J F et al., "Breaks in the wall: Increased gaps in the intestinal epithelium of irritable bowel syndrome patients identified by confocal laser endomicroscopy (with videos)", *Gastrointestinal Endoscopy*, 77(4), 2013, pp.624–630. doi: 10.1016/j.gie.2012.11.006. Epub 2013 Jan 26. PMID: 23357497

12 Camilleri, M et al., "Intestinal barrier function in health and gastrointestinal disease", *Neurogastroenterology & Motility*, 24(6), 2012, pp.503–512. doi: 10.1111/j.1365-2982.2012.01921.x. Erratum in: *Neurogastroenterology & Motility*, 24(10), 2012, p.976. Van Meerveld, B G [corrected to Greenwood-Van Meerveld, B]. PMID: 22583600; PMCID: PMC5595063

13 Hamer, H M et al., "Review article: The role of butyrate on colonic function", *Alimentary Pharmacology & Therapeutics*, 27(2), 2008, pp.104–119. doi: 10.1111/j.1365-2036.2007.03562.x. Epub 25 October 2007. PMID: 17973645

14 Chlebicz-Wójcik, A and Śliżewska, K, "Probiotics, prebiotics, and synbiotics in the irritable bowel syndrome treatment: A review", *Biomolecules*, 11, 2021, p.1154. doi.org/10.3390/biom11081154

15 Frost, G et al., "The short-chain fatty acid acetate reduces appetite via a central homeostatic mechanism", *Nature Communications*, 5(3611), 2014. doi.org/10.1038/ncomms4611

16 De Pessemier, B et al., "Gut–skin axis: Current knowledge of the interrelationship between microbial dysbiosis and skin conditions", *Microorganisms*, 9(2), 2021, p.353. doi: 10.3390/microorganisms9020353. PMID: 33670115; PMCID: PMC7916842

17 De Giorgio, R, Volta, U and Gibson, P R, "Sensitivity to wheat, gluten and FODMAPs in IBS: Facts or fiction?", *Gut*, 65, 2016, pp.169–178

18 Wang Jinsheng et al., "Low-FODMAP diet improves the global symptoms and bowel habits of adult IBS patients: A systematic review and meta-analysis", *Frontiers in Nutrition*, 8, 2021. doi: 10.3389/fnut.2021.683191

19 El-Salhy, M and Gundersen, D, "Diet in irritable bowel syndrome", *Nutrition Journal*, 14(1), 2015. doi.org/10.1186/s12937-015-0022-3

20 Tuck, C J et al., "Food intolerances", *Nutrients*, 11, 2019. doi.org/10.3390/nu11071684

21 Urwin, H et al., "Early recognition of coeliac disease through community pharmacies: A proof of concept study", *International Journal of Clinical Pharmacy*, 38(5), 2016, pp.1294–1300. doi: 10.1007/s11096-016-0368-4. Epub 2016 Aug 8. PMID: 27503280; PMCID: PMC5031749

22 Anon, Rostami, K and Hogg-Kollars, S, "Non-coeliac gluten sensitivity", *BMJ*, 2012. doi: 10.1136/bmj.e7982

23 https://www.mdpi.com/2072-6643/7/3/1565

24 https://www.mdpi.com/2072-6643/13/1/27

25 www.med.monash.edu

26 Sia, T et al., "Fructose malabsorption and fructan malabsorption are associated in patients with irritable bowel syndrome", *BMC Gastroenterology*, 24, 2024. doi.org/10.1186/s12876-024-03230-x

27 Kvehaugen, A S, Tveiten, D and Farup, P G, "Is perceived intolerance to milk and wheat associated with the corresponding IgG and IgA food antibodies? A cross sectional study in subjects with morbid obesity and gastrointestinal symptoms", *BMC Gastroenterology*, 18, 2018. doi.org/10.1186/s12876-018-0750-x

28 Benardout, M et al., "Fructose malabsorption: Causes, diagnosis and treatment", *British Journal of Nutrition*, 127(4), 2022, pp.481–489. doi: 10.1017/S0007114521001215

29 Reding, K W et al., "Relationship between patterns of alcohol consumption and gastrointestinal symptoms among patients with irritable bowel syndrome", *American Journal of Gastroenterology*, 108(2), 2013, pp.270–276. doi: 10.1038/ajg.2012.414. Epub 8 January 2013. PMID: 23295280; PMCID: PMC3697482

30 Ibid

31 Simrén, M et al., "Food-related gastrointestinal symptoms in the irritable bowel syndrome", *Digestion*, 63(2), 2001, pp.108–115. doi: 10.1159/000051878. PMID: 11244249

32 Vasant, D H et al., "British Society of Gastroenterology guidelines on the management of irritable bowel syndrome", *Gut*, 70, 2021, pp.1214–1240

33 Shulpekova, Y O et al., "Food intolerance: The role of histamine", *Nutrients*, 13, 2021. doi.org/10.3390/nu13093207

34 Hrubisko, M et al., "Histamine intolerance: The more we know the less we know: A review," *Nutrients*, 13, 2012. doi.org/10.3390/nu13072228

35 Sánchez-Pérez, S et al., "The dietary treatment of histamine intolerance reduces the abundance of some histamine-secreting bacteria of the gut microbiota in histamine intolerant women: A pilot study", *Frontiers in Nutrition*, 9, 2022. doi: 10.3389/fnut.2022.1018463

36 Schnedl, W J and Enko, D, "Histamine intolerance originates in the gut", *Nutrients*, 13, 2021. doi.org/10.3390/nu13041262

37 Borghini, R et al., "New insights in IBS-like disorders: Pandora's box has been opened. A review", *Gastroenterology and Hepatology From Bed to Bench*, 10(2), 2017, pp.79–89. PMID: 28702130; PMCID: PMC5495893

38 Kamerud, K L, Hobbie, K A and Anderson, K A, "Stainless steel leaches nickel and chromium into foods during cooking", *Journal of Agricultural and Food Chemistry*, 61(39), 2013, pp.9495–9501. doi: 10.1021/jf402400v. Epub 2013 Sep 19. PMID: 23984718; PMCID: PMC4284091

39 www.functionalmedicine.org

40 Karantanos, T et al., "Current insights in to the pathophysiology of irritable bowel syndrome," *Gut Pathogens*, 2, 2010. doi.org/10.1186/1757-4749-2-3

41 Antonelli, M and Donelli, D, "Kiwifruit (*Actinidia* spp.) dietary consumption for constipation: A systematic review and meta-analysis", *Future Pharmacology*, 1, 2021, pp.27–40. doi.org/10.3390/futurepharmacol1010003

42 Xu, J et al., "Laxative effects of partially defatted flaxseed meal on normal and experimental constipated mice", *BMC Complementary and Alternative Medicine*, 12(14), 2012. doi.org/10.1186/1472-6882-12-14

43 "A rice based diet with green banana or pectin reduced diarrhoea in infants better than a rice alone diet", *BMJ Evidence-Based Medicine*, 7(55), 2002

44 Wedlake, L et al., "Systematic review: The prevalence of idiopathic bile acid malabsorption as diagnosed by SeHCAT scanning in patients with diarrhoea-predominant irritable bowel syndrome", *Alimentary Pharmacology & Therapeutics*, 30(7), 2009, pp.707–717. doi: 10.1111/j.1365-2036.2009.04081.x. Epub 30 June 2009. PMID: 19570102

45 Fan, X and Sellin, J H, "Review article: Small intestinal bacterial overgrowth, bile acid malabsorption and gluten intolerance as possible causes of chronic watery diarrhoea", *Alimentary Pharmacology & Therapeutics*, 29(10), 2009, pp.1069–1077. doi: 10.1111/j.1365-2036.2009.03970.x. Epub 15 February 2009. Erratum in: *Alimentary Pharmacology & Therapeutics*, 29(11), 2009, p.1217. PMID: 19222407

46 Coffin, B et al., "Efficacy of a simethicone, activated charcoal and magnesium oxide combination (Carbosymag®) in functional dyspepsia: Results of a general practice-based randomized trial", *Clinics and Research in Hepatology and Gastroenterology*, 35(6–7), 2011, pp.494–499. doi: 10.1016/j.clinre.2011.02.009. Epub 7 April 2011. PMID: 21478070

47 Li Bing et al., "Efficacy and safety of probiotics in irritable bowel syndrome: A systematic review and meta-analysis", *Frontiers in Pharmacology*, 11, 2020. doi: 10.3389/fphar.2020.00332

48 Ringel-Kulka, T et al., "Probiotic bacteria *Lactobacillus acidophilus* NCFM and *Bifidobacterium lactis* Bi-07 versus placebo for the symptoms of bloating in patients with functional bowel disorders: A double-blind study", *Journal of Clinical Gastroenterology*, 45(6), 2011, pp.518–525. doi: 10.1097/MCG.0b013e31820ca4d6. PMID: 21436726; PMCID: PMC4372813

49 Whorwell, P J et al., "Efficacy of an encapsulated probiotic *Bifidobacterium infantis* 35624 in women with irritable bowel syndrome", *American Journal of Gastroenterology*, 101(7), 2006, pp.1581–1590

50 Ullah, H et al., "Efficacy of digestive enzyme supplementation in functional dyspepsia: A monocentric, randomized, double-blind, placebo-controlled, clinical trial", *Biomedicine & Pharmacotherapy*, 169, 2023. doi: 10.1016/j.biopha.2023.115858. Epub 14 November 2023. PMID: 37976892

51 Misselwitz, B et al., "Lactose malabsorption and intolerance: Pathogenesis, diagnosis and treatment", *United European Gastroenterology Journal*, 1(3), 2013, pp.151–159. doi: 10.1177/2050640613484463. PMID: 24917953; PMCID: PMC4040760

52 McMullen, M K et al., "Bitters: Time for a new paradigm", *Evidence-Based Complementary and Alternative Medicine*, 2015. doi.org/10.1155/2015/670504

53 Anh, N H et al., "Ginger on human health: A comprehensive systematic review of 109 randomized controlled trials", *Nutrients*, 12, 2020. doi.org/10.3390/nu12010157

54 Mao, Q.-Q et al., "Bioactive compounds and bioactivities of ginger (*Zingiber officinale* Roscoe)", *Foods*, 8, 2019. doi.org/10.3390/foods8060185

55 Foster Joy, J and Haber, S L, "Clinical uses of artichoke leaf extract", *American Journal of Health-System Pharmacy*, 64(18), 2007, pp.1904–1909. doi.org/10.2146/ajhp070013

56 Chao, H-C, "Zinc deficiency and therapeutic value of zinc supplementation in pediatric gastrointestinal diseases", *Nutrients*, 15(19), 2023. doi.org/10.3390/nu15194093

57 Mar-Solís, L M et al., "Analysis of the anti-inflammatory capacity of bone broth in a murine model of ulcerative colitis", *Medicina*, 57(11), 2021. doi.org/10.3390/medicina57111138

58 Xing, L et al., "The anti-inflammatory effect of bovine bone-gelatin-derived peptides in LPS-induced RAW264.7 macrophages cells and dextran sulfate sodium-induced C57BL/6 mice", *Nutrients*, 14(7), 2022. doi: 10.3390/nu14071479. PMID: 35406093; PMCID: PMC9003490

59 Abrahams, M, O'Grady, R and Prawitt, J, "Effect of a daily collagen peptide supplement on digestive symptoms in healthy women: 2-phase mixed methods study", *JMIR Formative Research*, 6(5), 2022. doi: 10.2196/36339. PMID: 35639457; PMCID: PMC9198822

60 Kim, M-H and Kim, H, "The roles of glutamine in the intestine and its implication in intestinal diseases", *International Journal of Molecular Sciences*, 18, 2017. doi.org/10.3390/ijms18051051

61 Suzuki, T and Hara, H, "Quercetin enhances intestinal barrier function through the assembly of zonnula occludens-2, occludin, and claudin-1 and the expression of claudin-4 in caco-2 cells", *Journal of Nutrition*, 139(5), 2009, pp.965–974

62 Hou, Y et al., "N-acetylcysteine and intestinal health: A focus on mechanisms of its actions", *Frontiers in Bioscience* (Landmark edition), 20, 2015, pp.872–891

63 Bodammer, P et al., "Bovine colostrum increases pore-forming claudin-2 protein expression but paradoxically not ion permeability possibly by a change of the intestinal cytokine milieu", *PLoS ONE*, 8(5), 2013. doi: 10.1371/journal.pone.0064210. PMID: 23717570; PMCID: PMC3662709

64 Graham, M F et al., "Collagen synthesis by human intestinal smooth muscle cells in culture", *Gastroenterology*, 92(2), 1987, pp.400–405. doi: 10.1016/0016-5085(87)90134-x. PMID: 3792777

65 Hui Yan and Ajuwon, K M, "Butyrate modifies intestinal barrier function in IPEC-J2 cells through a selective upregulation of tight junction proteins and activation of the Akt signaling pathway", *PLoS ONE*, 12(6), 2017. doi.org/10.1371/journal.pone.0179586

66 Hilimire M R, DeVylder J E, Forestell C A, "Fermented foods, neuroticism, and social anxiety: An interaction model", *Psychiatry Res*, 228(2), 2015, pp. 203-8. doi: 10.1016/j.psychres.2015.04.023. Epub 28 April 2015. PMID: 25998000.

67 Johannesson, E et al., "Physical activity improves symptoms in irritable bowel syndrome: A randomized controlled trial", *American Journal of Gastroenterology*,

106(5), 2011, pp.915–922. doi: 10.1038/ajg.2010.480. Epub 2011 Jan 4. PMID: 21206488

68 D'Silva, A et al., "Meditation and yoga for irritable bowel syndrome: A randomized clinical trial", *American Journal of Gastroenterology*, 118(2), 2023, pp.329–337. doi: 10.14309/ajg.0000000000002052. Epub 2022 Oct 11. PMID: 36422517; PMCID: PMC9889201

69 Bilski, J et al., "The role of physical exercise in inflammatory bowel disease", *BioMed Research International*, 2014(1), 2014. doi: 10.1155/2014/429031. Epub 2014 Apr 30. PMID: 24877092; PMCID: PMC4022156

70 Hosseini-Asl, M K, Taherifard, E and Mousavi, M R, "The effect of a short-term physical activity after meals on gastrointestinal symptoms in individuals with functional abdominal bloating: A randomized clinical trial", *Gastroenterology and Hepatology From Bed to Bench*, 14(1), 2021, pp.59–66. PMID: 33868611; PMCID: PMC8035544

71 Johannesson, E et al., "Intervention to increase physical activity in irritable bowel syndrome shows long-term positive effects", *World Journal of Gastroenterology*, 21(2), 2015, pp.600–608. doi: 10.3748/wjg.v21.i2.600. PMID: 25593485; PMCID: PMC4294172

72 Tu, Q et al., "Sleep disturbances in irritable bowel syndrome: A systematic review", *Neurogastroenterology & Motility*, 29(3), 2017. doi: 10.1111/nmo.12946. Epub 28 September 2016. PMID: 27683238

73 Lu, W Z et al., "Melatonin improves bowel symptoms in female patients with irritable bowel syndrome: A double-blind placebo-controlled study", *Alimentary Pharmacology & Therapeutics*, 22(10), 2005, pp.927–934. doi: 10.1111/j.1365-2036.2005.02673.x. PMID: 16268966

74 Paduano, D et al., "Effect of three diets (low-FODMAP, gluten-free and balanced) on irritable bowel syndrome symptoms and health-related quality of life", *Nutrients*, 11(7), 2019. doi: 10.3390/nu11071566. PMID: 31336747; PMCID: PMC6683324

75 Nielsen, E S et al., "Lacto-fermented sauerkraut improves symptoms in IBS patients independent of product pasteurisation: A pilot study", *Food & Function*, 9(10), 2018, pp.5323–5335. doi: 10.1039/c8fo00968f. PMID: 30256365

76 Wastyk, H C et al., "Gut-microbiota-targeted diets modulate human immune status", *Cell*, 184(16), 2021, pp.4137–4153.e14. doi: 10.1016/j.cell.2021.06.019. Epub 12 July 2021. PMID: 34256014; PMCID: PMC9020749

77 Gayoso, L et al., "The effect of starch- and sucrose-reduced diet accompanied by nutritional and culinary recommendations on the symptoms of irritable bowel syndrome patients with diarrhoea", *Therapeutic Advances in Gastroenterology*, 16, 2023. doi: 10.1177/17562848231156682. PMID: 37153501; PMCID: PMC10155021

78 Nilholm, C et al., "A starch- and sucrose-reduced dietary intervention in irritable bowel syndrome patients produced a shift in gut microbiota composition along with changes in phylum, genus, and amplicon sequence variant abundances, without affecting the micro-RNA levels", *United European Gastroenterology Journal*, 10(4), 2022, pp.363–375. doi: 10.1002/ueg2.12227. Epub 2022 Apr 28. PMID: 35484927; PMCID: PMC9103372

79 Wilder-Smith, C H, Materna, A and Olesen, S S, "Blueberries improve abdominal symptoms, well-being and functioning in patients with functional gastrointestinal disorders", *Nutrients*, 15(10), 2023. doi.org/10.3390/nu15102396

Index

NUMBERS

5R approach, 12, 18–36
   basic recipes, 37–55
   example programme, 32–6

A

acetate, 9, 14
acid, stomach. *See* stomach acid
acid reflux, 5, 7, 19
acne, 9
activated charcoal, 21
agar flakes, 144
aioli, Grilled Prawns with Turmeric
   Lemon Aioli, 106–7
alcohol, 9, 13–14, 19, 20, 29
allergies, 10, 19
almond flour, Spinach, Tomato & Red
   Pepper Almond-Crusted Quiche,
   138–9
almonds, 11
   Almond Milk, 40
   Almond Yogurt, 47
   Baked Chicken with Barbecue
     Sauce, 116–17
   Blueberry Almond Bread, 64–5
   Breakfast Seed Bars, 67
   Broccoli Pizza, 96–7
   Caramel Apple Chia Pots, 70–1
   Fennel & Poppy-Seed Crispbreads,
     164–5
   Granola Fruit Bowl, 141
   Mocha Swirl Cheesecake, 150–1
   Paleo Carrot & Ginger Cake, 158–9
   Pumpkin & Cinnamon Paleo
     Granola, 68–9
   Raw Mango, Turmeric & Cardamom
     Tart, 154

Raw Orange Brownie Slices, 155
Raw Pad Thai with Courgette &
   Carrot Noodles, 108
Seeded Paleo Bread, 66
American Gut Project, 14–15
amino acids, 23, 24, 37, 44, 98, 114,
   117
   Asian Coconut Broth with Prawn
     Dumplings, 90–1
   glutamine, 61
   Matcha Green Tea & Lemon
     Breakfast Muffins, 62–3
   Pomegranate Lamb Tagine with
     Cauliflower Rice, 124–5
anchovies, Cod with Mediterranean
   Herb Dressing, 129
antibiotics, and IBS, 7
anti-inflammatory foods, 30, 114, 130,
   143, 150
   See also fats, omega-3
antioxidants, 39, 109, 114, 130, 144
   5R approach, 23–4, 30
   green tea, 64
   nuts, 151
anxiety, 64
   See also stress
apple cider vinegar, 37, 119, 135
   Barbecue Kale Crisps, 169
   Beetroot Cumin Crisps, 170–1
apples, 17, 24, 30
   Apple & Plum Crisp, 152–3
   Baked Chicken with Barbecue
     Sauce, 116–17
   Caramel Apple Chia Pots, 70–1
   Light Digestive Lemon Aid, 58
   Smoked Salmon with Sweet Potato
     Apple Röstis, 76–7

Spiced Roasted Beetroot & Apple
   Soup, 88–9
apricots, 13, 20
   Pomegranate Lamb Tagine with
     Cauliflower Rice, 124–5
artichokes, 22
   Chicken & Artichoke Salad with
     Roasted Garlic & Herb Dressing, 93
artificial sweeteners, 29
Asian Coconut Broth with Prawn
   Dumplings, 90–1
Asian-Spiced Lettuce Wraps, 94–5
astaxanthin, 107
autoimmune disorders, 7
   See also coeliac disease
avocados
   Chipotle Avocado Cream Spread,
     168
   Cumin-Spiced Halibut with Kale
     Salad, 132–3
   Lime-Marinated Salmon Salad with
     Fennel & Mango, 101
   Mint & Chocolate Ice, 140
   Vegan Mexican Taco Bowl, 136

B

bacon, Vietnamese Prawn & Bacon
   Fried "Rice," 132–3
bacteria
   beneficial, 22, 24, 25, 29, 144
   See also gut microbes/bacteria
Baked Chicken with Barbecue Sauce,
   116–17
balsamic vinegar
   Baked Chicken with Barbecue
     Sauce, 116–17
   Harissa Roasted Tofu Salad, 110

balsamic vinegar (*continued*)
Lentil & Goat's Cheese Salad with
Roasted Red Peppers, 111
Southern-Spiced Pulled Pork with
Sauerkraut, 119
bananas, 17, 20, 25
Blueberry Almond Bread, 66–7
Granola Fruit Bowl, 141
Green Gut Healer, 61
Barbecue Kale Crisps, 169
basil, Asian-Spiced Lettuce Wraps,
94–5
beans and pulses
beneficial bacteria, 23
and fructans, 11–12, 29
Lentil & Goat's Cheese Salad with
Roasted Red Peppers, 111
Mandarin Salad of Duck with Green
Beans, 120
beef
Beef & Liver Burgers with Wasabi
Mayo, 128
bone broth, 37
Korean Spiced Beef with Kimchi,
124–5
Purple-Sprouting Broccoli & Beef
Kelp Noodle Salad, 100
beetroot/beets, 22, 30
Beetroot Cumin Crisps, 170–1
Red Cabbage and Beetroot
Sauerkraut, 53
Spiced Roasted Beetroot & Apple
Soup, 88–9
berries, 17, 24
Antioxidant Blast, 63
Buttermilk Waffles with Berries, 74
Cherry & Coconut Layered Parfait,
144–5
Chocolate Maca Cream, 63
Cumin-Spiced Halibut with Kale
Salad, 132–3
Granola Fruit Bowl, 141
Lemon Balm & Berry Ice, 140

Pan-Seared Venison with
Blueberries & Broccoli Mash,
122–3
and polyphenols, 30
betalains, 166
Bifidobacterium species, 11
bile, 20, 22, 88, 166
bitter greens, 21
See also rocket/arugula; watercress
blinis and pancakes, Fluffy Coconut
Blinis with Spiced Fruit Compote,
74–5
bloating, 5, 12, 19, 21, 23, 160
blueberries, 30
Blueberry Almond Bread, 66–7
Pan-Seared Venison with
Blueberries & Broccoli Mash,
122–3
bone broth, 23, 37
Asian Coconut Broth with Prawn
Dumplings, 90–1
Braised Chicken with Green Olives
& Preserved Lemon, 114–15
Pan-Seared Venison with
Blueberries & Broccoli Mash,
122–3
Spiced Roasted Beetroot & Apple
Soup, 88–9
box breathing, 25
brain health, 14
Braised Chicken with Green Olives &
Preserved Lemon, 112–13
Breakfast Seed Bars, 69
breathing techniques, 25
British Society of Gastroenterology, 14
broccoli
Broccoli & Watercress Cleanse, 92
Broccoli Pizza, 96–7
Korean Spiced Beef with Kimchi,
124–5
Pan-Seared Venison with
Blueberries & Broccoli Mash,
122–3

Purple-Sprouting Broccoli & Beef
Kelp Noodle Salad, 100
butter, 12
Buttermilk Waffles with Berries, 74
butternut squash, 30
Pomegranate Lamb Tagine with
Cauliflower Rice, 124–5
butyrate, 9, 14, 24, 38

C
cabbage
Red Cabbage and Beetroot
Sauerkraut, 53
Sauerkraut, 52
Speedy Kimchi, 54
cacao butter
Matcha Superfood Bites, 160–1
Raw Mango, Turmeric & Cardamom
Tart, 150
cacao powder, 24
Chocolate Maca Cream, 63
Matcha Superfood Bites, 156–7
Mocha Swirl Cheesecake, 150–1
Raw Orange Brownie Slices, 155
caffeine, 14, 20, 26, 29
cakes
Paleo Carrot & Ginger Cake, 158–9
See also cheesecakes
calcium, 37, 44
candies, Fruity Gummy Sweets, 159
capers, Cod with Mediterranean Herb
Dressing, 129
Caramel Apple Chia Pots, 70–1
carbohydrates, 18, 29
See also FODMAPs
cardamom, Raw Mango, Turmeric &
Cardamom Tart, 150
carrots, 30
Paleo Carrot & Ginger Cake, 158–9
Purple-Sprouting Broccoli & Beef
Kelp Noodle Salad, 100
Raw Pad Thai with Courgette &
Carrot Noodles, 108

Sauerkraut, 52
Tempeh & Mushroom Bolognese, 140
Tofu Rice Bowl with Miso-Lemon Dressing, 139
cashew nuts, 28, 39
Broccoli & Watercress Cleanse, 92
Fennel & Poppy-Seed Crispbreads, 160–1
Lemon Balm & Berry Ice, 140
Lentil & Goat's Cheese Salad with Roasted Red Peppers, 111
Mocha Swirl Cheesecake, 150–1
Raw Herb Cashew Cheese, 49
Raw Mango, Turmeric & Cardamom Tart, 150
Raw Pad Thai with Courgette & Carrot Noodles, 108
Vegan Mexican Taco Bowl, 136
Vegan Nut Cream, 48
cauliflower
Crispy Cauliflower Popcorn, 168–9
Pomegranate Lamb Tagine with Cauliflower Rice, 124–5
Sicilian Tabbouleh with Cauliflower Rice, 109
Vietnamese Prawn & Bacon Fried "Rice," 134–5
cayenne pepper, 126
celery
Lebanese Lamb Salad, 98–9
Restorative Chicken Noodle Soup, 86–7
Tempeh & Mushroom Bolognese, 140
cheese
Broccoli Pizza, 96–7
hard, low lactose, 12
cheesecakes, Mocha Swirl Cheesecake, 150–1
cherries, 30, 159
Cherry & Coconut Layered Parfait, 144–5

Matcha Superfood Bites, 160–1
chia, 28
chia seeds, 63
Caramel Apple Chia Pots, 70–1
Chia, Flaxseed & Tomato Crackers, 162–3
Lemon Cream Sandwich Cookies, 156–7
Matcha Green Tea & Lemon Breakfast Muffins, 62–3
chicken
Baked Chicken with Barbecue Sauce, 116–17
bone broth, 37, 91
Braised Chicken with Green Olives & Preserved Lemon, 114–15
Chicken & Artichoke Salad with Roasted Garlic & Herb Dressing, 93
Restorative Chicken Noodle Soup, 86–7
chicken livers
Beef & Liver Burgers with Wasabi Mayo, 128
Pan-Fried Indian-Spiced Liver, 77
chillies
Asian-Spiced Lettuce Wraps, 94–5
Grilled Prawns with Turmeric Lemon Aioli, 106–7
Korean Spiced Beef with Kimchi, 124–5
Lime-Marinated Salmon Salad with Fennel & Mango, 101
Purple-Sprouting Broccoli & Beef Kelp Noodle Salad, 100
Restorative Chicken Noodle Soup, 86–7
Tempeh & Mushroom Bolognese, 140
Vegan Mexican Taco Bowl, 136
Vietnamese Prawn & Bacon Fried "Rice," 134–5
Chipotle Avocado Cream Spread, 168

chives, Spinach, Tomato & Red Pepper Almond-Crusted Quiche, 138–9
chocolate, 19
Chocolate Bounty Bites, 162
Chocolate Maca Cream, 63
Mint & Chocolate Ice, 140
cinnamon
Apple & Plum Crisp, 152–3
Fluffy Coconut Blinis with Spiced Fruit Compote, 74–5
Granola Fruit Bowl, 141
Mandarin Salad of Duck with Green Beans, 120
Overnight Oats with Kiwi & Pomegranate, 84
Pumpkin & Cinnamon Paleo Granola, 70
citrus juice, 21
Citrus Mojito Kombucha, 58
coconut oil, 126, 150
Apple & Plum Crisp, 148–9
Blueberry Almond Bread, 66–7
Breakfast Seed Bars, 69
Chocolate Bounty Bites, 162
Lemon Cream Sandwich Cookies, 156–7
Lime-Marinated Salmon Salad with Fennel & Mango, 101
Raw Orange Brownie Slices, 155
Seeded Paleo Bread, 66
Sicilian Tabbouleh with Cauliflower Rice, 109
coconuts/coconut milks, 40, 41, 44
Antioxidant Blast, 63
Asian Coconut Broth with Prawn Dumplings, 90–1
Cherry & Coconut Layered Parfait, 144–5
Chocolate Bounty Bites, 158
Coconut Yogurt, 47
Creamy Turmeric Kefir, 61
Granola Fruit Bowl, 141
Lemon Balm & Berry Ice, 140

coconuts/coconut milks (*continued*)
  Matcha Green Tea & Lemon
    Breakfast Muffins, 62–3
  Mint & Chocolate Ice, 140
  Mocha Swirl Cheesecake, 150–1
  Paleo Carrot & Ginger Cake, 158–9
  Pan-Seared Venison with Blueberries
    & Broccoli Mash, 122–3
  Pumpkin & Cinnamon Paleo
    Granola, 70
  Raw Mango, Turmeric & Cardamom
    Tart, 150
  Spinach, Tomato & Red Pepper
    Almond-Crusted Quiche, 138–9
  Tropical Fruit Platter with Sweet
    Ginger & Mint Dressing, 146–7
  See also flour, coconut
Cod with Mediterranean Herb
  Dressing, 128–9
coeliac disease, 7, 10, 13, 22, 27
coffee, 19, 29, 30
  Mocha Swirl Cheesecake, 150–1
collagen, 24, 31
  Chocolate Bounty Bites, 162
colostrum, 24, 31
constipation, 7, 10
  and caffeine, 14
  easing, 19–20
  IBS-C, 5
  supplements, 31
cookies, Lemon Cream Sandwich
  Cookies, 156–7
coriander
  Asian Coconut Broth with Prawn
    Dumplings, 90–1
  Asian-Spiced Lettuce Wraps, 94–5
  Chipotle Avocado Cream Spread,
    168
  Light Digestive Lemon Aid, 58
  Lime-Marinated Salmon Salad with
    Fennel & Mango, 101
  Restorative Chicken Noodle Soup,
    86–7

Roasted Whole Salmon with Sweet
  Soy & Star Anise, 127
Spiced Omelette, 80–1
cortisol (stress hormone), 25, 26
courgette/zucchini
  Hot-Smoked Trout with Pistachio
    Pesto Noodles, 102–3
  Raw Pad Thai with Courgette &
    Carrot Noodles, 108
  Restorative Chicken Noodle Soup,
    86–7
  Turkey Meatballs with Roasted
    Tomato Chipotle Sauce, 118–19
crackers and crispbreads
  Chia, Flaxseed & Tomato Crackers,
    162–3
  Fennel & Poppy-Seed Crispbreads,
    160–1
Creamy Turmeric Kefir, 61
crispbreads and crackers. *See* crackers
  and crispbreads
crisps, vegetable
  Barbecue Kale Crisps, 169
  Beetroot Cumin Crisps, 170–1
Crohn's disease, 8, 12
cucumbers
  Lebanese Lamb Salad, 98–9
  Light Digestive Lemon Aid, 58
  Pickled Dill Cucumber, 51
  Sicilian Tabbouleh with Cauliflower
    Rice, 109
cumin seeds/ground cumin
  Beetroot Cumin Crisps, 170–1
  Cumin-Spiced Halibut with Kale
    Salad, 132–3
  Harissa Roasted Tofu Salad, 110
  Lebanese Lamb Salad, 98–9
  Pan-Fried Indian-Spiced Liver, 77
  Spiced Roasted Beetroot & Apple
    Soup, 88–9
  Sunflower Seed & Mushroom
    Falafels with Tahini Lemon
    Dressing, 135

D

dairy foods, 17, 27–8
  See also cheese; lactose; milk; yogurt
dandelion coffee, Mocha Swirl
  Cheesecake, 150–1
dates
  Barbecue Kale Crisps, 169
  Breakfast Seed Bars, 69
  Caramel Apple Chia Pots, 70–1
  Mocha Swirl Cheesecake, 150–1
  Paleo Carrot & Ginger Cake, 158–9
  Raw Orange Brownie Slices, 155
  Sunflower Seed & Mushroom
    Falafels with Tahini Lemon
    Dressing, 135
diamine oxidase (DAO), 15
diarrhoea, 10
  bananas for, 141
  food irritants, 19
  and IBS, 5, 6, 7
  and lactose intolerance, 12
  supplements, 31
  symptoms, understanding and
    managing, 20–1
diets
  FODMAPs. *See* FODMAPs
  Western-style, and IBS, 7
  and your gut microbes, 9
digestive enzymes, 30
dragon fruit, Tropical Fruit Platter with
  Sweet Ginger & Mint Dressing, 146–7
dried fruit, 25
  Raw Mango, Turmeric & Cardamom
    Tart, 150
duck, Mandarin Salad of Duck with
  Green Beans, 120
dukka, Poached Eggs with Wilted Kale,
  Tomato & Dukka, 82–3
dysbiosis, 6–7, 19, 25

E

eczema, 9, 15
eggs

Baked Chicken with Barbecue Sauce, 116–17

Beef & Liver Burgers with Wasabi Mayo, 128

Blueberry Almond Bread, 66–7

Broccoli Pizza, 96–7

Fluffy Coconut Blinis with Spiced Fruit Compote, 74–5

Matcha Green Tea & Lemon Breakfast Muffins, 62–3

mayonnaise, 39

Paleo Carrot & Ginger Cake, 158–9

Poached Eggs with Wilted Kale, Tomato & Dukka, 82–3

Spiced Omelette, 80–1

Spinach, Tomato & Red Pepper Almond-Crusted Quiche, 138–9

Vietnamese Prawn & Bacon Fried "Rice," 132–3

enteric nervous system, 8

enzymes, 8, 15, 21

exercise, physical, 9, 18, 21, 25–6

F

falafels, Sunflower Seed & Mushroom Falafels with Tahini Lemon Dressing, 135

fats

    anti-inflammatory foods, 39, 70

    malabsorption of, 7

    omega-3, 91, 101, 103, 107, 127, 129, 130

    omega-3 and -9, 24, 38

    as part of healthy diet, 28, 30

fatty acids, 98

fennel bulb

    Light Digestive Lemon Aid, 58

    Lime-Marinated Salmon Salad with Fennel & Mango, 101

fennel seeds, Fennel & Poppy-Seed Crispbreads, 160–1

fermentable fibres (GOS), 28

fermented foods, 9, 17, 20, 22, 29, 42–9

grains, 22

kefir, 44–5

Kombucha. See kombucha

Raw Herb Cashew Cheese, 49

Vegan Nut Cream, 48

yogurt, 46–7

See also pickles

fibre

    and bloating, 21

    breakfasts, 84

    fructans, 28

    and general health, 14–15

    and IBS, 14, 20

    insoluble, 14

    and prebiotics, 23

    seeds for, 153

    soluble, 14, 141, 148

fish

    oily fish, 24

    protein, 24

    See also prawns/shrimps; specific fish

fish oils, 31

fish sauce

    Lime-Marinated Salmon Salad with Fennel & Mango, 101

    Purple-Sprouting Broccoli & Beef Kelp Noodle Salad, 100

flaxseed oil, Sicilian Tabbouleh with Cauliflower Rice, 109

flaxseeds, 21, 28, 39

    Buttermilk Waffles with Berries, 74

    Chia, Flaxseed & Tomato Crackers, 162–3

    Seeded Paleo Bread, 66

flour, coconut

    Broccoli Pizza, 96–7

    Fluffy Coconut Blinis with Spiced Fruit Compote, 74–5

    Lemon Cream Sandwich Cookies, 156–7

    Matcha Green Tea & Lemon Breakfast Muffins, 62–3

Paleo Carrot & Ginger Cake, 154–5

Fluffy Coconut Blinis with Spiced Fruit Compote, 74–5

FODMAPs

    and bloating, 21

    low FODMAP diet, 118

    prebiotics and, 17

    reducing or removing, 19

    understanding, 11–15

food allergies/intolerances, 10, 19

food poisoning, and IBS, 6

fried and fatty foods, 19, 21

    See also fats

fructans, 10, 11–12, 23, 28–9, 87

fructose, 11, 13, 28, 29

fruit juices, 28

Fruity Gummy Sweets, 159

functional bowel disorders, 4

functional dyspepsia, 21

G

garlic

    Asian-Spiced Lettuce Wraps, 94–5

    Braised Chicken with Green Olives & Preserved Lemon, 115

    Chicken & Artichoke Salad with Roasted Garlic & Herb Dressing, 93

    Mandarin Salad of Duck with Green Beans, 120

    Poached Eggs with Wilted Kale, Tomato & Dukka, 82–3

    Pomegranate Lamb Tagine with Cauliflower Rice, 124–5

    Purple-Sprouting Broccoli & Beef Kelp Noodle Salad, 100

    Roasted Whole Salmon with Sweet Soy & Star Anise, 127

    Tempeh & Mushroom Bolognese, 140

    Vegan Mexican Taco Bowl, 136

gastric mucosa, 22

gelatine, 23, 37
   Cherry & Coconut Layered Parfait, 144–5
   Fruity Gummy Sweets, 159
ghee, 38
Giardia, 6
ginger, 22, 24
   Asian Coconut Broth with Prawn Dumplings, 90–1
   Baked Chicken with Barbecue Sauce, 116–17
   Korean Spiced Beef with Kimchi, 124–5
   Paleo Carrot & Ginger Cake, 158–9
   Pan-Fried Indian-Spiced Liver, 77
   Pomegranate Lamb Tagine with Cauliflower Rice, 122–3
   Purple-Sprouting Broccoli & Beef Kelp Noodle Salad, 100
   Roasted Whole Salmon with Sweet Soy & Star Anise, 127
   Tamarind-Glazed Mackerel, 104–5
tea, 21
   Tofu Rice Bowl with Miso-Lemon Dressing, 139
   Tropical Fruit Platter with Sweet Ginger & Mint Dressing, 146–7
   Turmeric-Infused Daikon, Red Radish & Ginger Pickle, 55
   Vietnamese Prawn & Bacon Fried "Rice," 134–5
globe artichokes. See artichokes
glutamine, 23, 31, 61
gluten, problems with, 10
gluten-free foods
   Fluffy Coconut Blinis with Spiced Fruit Compote, 74
   Seeded Paleo Bread, 66
goat's cheese, Lentil & Goat's Cheese Salad with Roasted Red Peppers, 111
goji berries
   Cherry & Coconut Layered Parfait, 144–5

Cumin-Spiced Halibut with Kale Salad, 132–3
Granola Fruit Bowl, 141
Matcha Superfood Bites, 160–1
Paleo Carrot & Ginger Cake, 158–9
granola
   Granola Fruit Bowl, 141
   Pumpkin & Cinnamon Paleo Granola, 70, 141
green beans, Mandarin Salad of Duck with Green Beans, 120
Green Gut Healer, 61
green tea, 23, 25, 30, 43
   Matcha Green Tea & Lemon Breakfast Muffins, 62–3
   Matcha Superfood Bites, 160–1
   Mint & Chocolate Ice, 140
Grilled Prawns with Turmeric Lemon Aioli, 106–7
gut microbes/bacteria
   5R approach, 31
   beneficial, 22, 24, 29
   Bifidobacterium species, 11
   and IBS, 6–9
gut-brain axis, 8, 25

H

halibut, Cumin-Spiced Halibut with Kale Salad, 132–3
Harissa Roasted Tofu Salad, 110
hazelnuts
   Lentil & Goat's Cheese Salad with Roasted Red Peppers, 111
   Poached Eggs with Wilted Kale, Tomato & Dukka, 82–3
headaches, 5, 15
heartburn, 13, 22, 24
hemp oils, 28
herb dressings
   Chicken & Artichoke Salad with Roasted Garlic & Herb Dressing, 93
   Cod with Mediterranean Herb Dressing, 128–9

Sicilian Tabbouleh with Cauliflower Rice, 109
herbs
   Chicken & Artichoke Salad with Roasted Garlic & Herb Dressing, 93
   for gut dysbiosis/ gut infections, 19
   Sicilian Tabbouleh with Cauliflower Rice, 109
   smoothies, 24
   and stress, 25
   Vietnamese Prawn & Bacon Fried "Rice," 134–5
   See also specific herbs
histamine, 6, 15, 31
honey, 28, 29, 130
   Apple & Plum Crisp, 152–3
   Paleo Carrot & Ginger Cake, 158–9
horseradish, 22, 126
Hot-Smoked Trout with Pistachio Pesto Noodles, 102–3
hydrochloric acid, 21

I

ice cream
   Lemon Balm & Berry Ice, 140
   Mint & Chocolate Ice, 140
IgE antibody test, 10
immune system
   and allergies, 10
   digestive tract and, 18
   fibre and, 14
   gut-brain axis and, 8
   and IBS, 6–7
indigestion, chronic, 21
inflammation, 6, 7, 15, 25
Institute of Functional Medicine, 18
intestinal permeability, 7
intestines, lining of, 23
   See also small intestine
iron, 39, 85, 117
irritable bowel syndrome (IBS)
   5R approach, 19

artichoke for, 22

and exercise, 25

and fibre, 14

and FODMAPs, 11–12

and food reactions/triggers, 9–10, 14–16

and fructose, 13

IBS-C, 5

IBS-D, 5, 20

IBS-M, 5

IBS-U, 5

occurrence of, 4, 5

and sleep, 26

understanding, and causes of, 5–8

J

juniper berries, Pan-Seared Venison with Blueberries & Broccoli Mash, 122–3

K

kale

Barbecue Kale Crisps, 169

Cumin-Spiced Halibut with Kale Salad, 132–3

Green Gut Healer, 61

Poached Eggs with Wilted Kale, Tomato & Dukka, 82–3

kefir

Creamy Turmeric Kefir, 61

Fluffy Coconut Blinis with Spiced Fruit Compote, 74–5

Lemon Balm & Berry Ice, 140

Milk Kefir, 44

Raw Mango, Turmeric & Cardamom Tart, 150

Seeded Paleo Bread, 66

Water Kefir, 45

kelp noodles, Purple-Sprouting Broccoli & Beef Kelp Noodle Salad, 100

kimchi, 29

Korean Spiced Beef with Kimchi, 124–5

Speedy Kimchi, 54

Spiced Omelette, 80–1

kiwi fruit

Green Gut Healer, 61

Overnight Oats with Kiwi & Pomegranate, 84

kombucha, 43

Citrus Mojito Kombucha, 58

Fruity Gummy Sweets, 159

Raw Mango, Turmeric & Cardamom Tart, 150

Korean Spiced Beef with Kimchi, 124–5

L

lactose, 11, 12–13, 20, 27–8

lamb

Lebanese Lamb Salad, 98–9

Pomegranate Lamb Tagine with Cauliflower Rice, 122–3

leaky gut, 7, 23, 24

Lebanese Lamb Salad, 98–9

Lemon Balm & Berry Ice, 140

lemons

Braised Chicken with Green Olives & Preserved Lemon, 114–15

Broccoli & Watercress Cleanse, 92

Citrus Mojito Kombucha, 58

Cumin-Spiced Halibut with Kale Salad, 132–3

Fruity Gummy Sweets, 159

Grilled Prawns with Turmeric Lemon Aioli, 106–7

Lebanese Lamb Salad, 98–9

Lemon Balm & Berry Ice, 140

Lemon Cream Sandwich Cookies, 156–7

Matcha Green Tea & Lemon Breakfast Muffins, 62–3

Sicilian Tabbouleh with Cauliflower Rice, 109

Sunflower Seed & Mushroom Falafels with Tahini Lemon Dressing, 135

Tamarind-Glazed Mackerel, 104–5

Tofu Rice Bowl with Miso-Lemon Dressing, 139

Tropical Fruit Platter with Sweet Ginger & Mint Dressing, 146–7

lentils, 29

Lentil & Goat's Cheese Salad with Roasted Red Peppers, 111

lettuce

Asian-Spiced Lettuce Wraps, 94–5

Southern-Spiced Pulled Pork with Sauerkraut, 119

Vegan Mexican Taco Bowl, 136

See also salad

Light Digestive Lemon Aid, 58

limes

Asian-Spiced Lettuce Wraps, 94–5

Lime-Marinated Salmon Salad with Fennel & Mango, 101

Purple-Sprouting Broccoli & Beef Kelp Noodle Salad, 100

Spiced Roasted Beetroot & Apple Soup, 88–9

Turkey Meatballs with Roasted Tomato Chipotle Sauce, 118–19

Vietnamese Prawn & Bacon Fried "Rice," 134–5

liver

Pan-Fried Indian-Spiced Liver, 77

See also chicken livers

low FODMAP diet, and your gut microbes, 9

lucuma powder, 153

lychees, Tropical Fruit Platter with Sweet Ginger & Mint Dressing, 146–7

M

maca

Chocolate Maca Cream, 63

Granola Fruit Bowl, 141

macadamia nuts, Sunflower Seed & Mushroom Falafels with Tahini Lemon Dressing, 135 mackerel, Tamarind-Glazed Mackerel, 104–5

magnesium, 25, 37, 44, 148, 165
    nuts, 151
    Tofu Scramble, 85

Mandarin Salad of Duck with Green Beans, 120

mangos
    Lime-Marinated Salmon Salad with Fennel & Mango, 101
    Raw Mango, Turmeric & Cardamom Tart, 150

maple syrup, 29
    Chocolate Bounty Bites, 158
    Fluffy Coconut Blinis with Spiced Fruit Compote, 74–5
    Harissa Roasted Tofu Salad, 110
    Lemon Balm & Berry Ice, 140
    Mandarin Salad of Duck with Green Beans, 120
    Pumpkin & Cinnamon Paleo Granola, 70
    Roasted Whole Salmon with Sweet Soy & Star Anise, 127
    Tofu Rice Bowl with Miso-Lemon Dressing, 139
    Tropical Fruit Platter with Sweet Ginger & Mint Dressing, 146–7

mast cells, 6

Matcha Green Tea & Lemon Breakfast Muffins, 64–5
    Matcha Superfood Bites, 160–1

mayonnaise, 39
    Lebanese Lamb Salad, 98–9

meatballs, Turkey Meatballs with Roasted Tomato Chipotle Sauce, 118–19

meats
    Broccoli Pizza, 96–7
    broth. See bone broth
    protein, 24
    See also specific meats

medications and supplements, 19
    See also supplements

meditation, 25

melatonin, 26

mental health issues, 5, 10

metabolism, 14, 17

microbial infection, 30

milk
    colostrum, 24
    Milk Kefir, 44

mind–body therapies, 25

mindfulness, 25, 26

mint, 19
    Citrus Mojito Kombucha, 58
    Lebanese Lamb Salad, 98–9
    Lime-Marinated Salmon Salad with Fennel & Mango, 101
    Mint & Chocolate Ice, 140
    Spiced Roasted Beetroot & Apple Soup, 88–9
    Tropical Fruit Platter with Sweet Ginger & Mint Dressing, 146–7

miso/miso dressing, Tofu Rice Bowl with Miso-Lemon Dressing, 139
    Mocha Swirl Cheesecake, 150–1

mood/wellbeing, and IBS, 8

muffins, Matcha Green Tea & Lemon Breakfast Muffins, 64–5

mushrooms
    Korean Spiced Beef with Kimchi, 124–5
    Mandarin Salad of Duck with Green Beans, 120
    Pan-Fried Indian-Spiced Liver, 77
    polyols, 13
    Sunflower Seed & Mushroom Falafels with Tahini Lemon Dressing, 135
    Tempeh & Mushroom Bolognese, 140
    Tofu Rice Bowl with Miso-Lemon Dressing, 139
    Vietnamese Prawn & Bacon Fried "Rice," 134–5

mustard, 111, 119

N

N-acetyl-cysteine (NAC), 24

nickel sensitivity, 15–16

non-coeliac gluten sensitivity (NCGS), 10

noodles
    Hot-Smoked Trout with Pistachio Pesto Noodles, 102–3
    Purple-Sprouting Broccoli & Beef Kelp Noodle Salad, 100
    Raw Pad Thai with Courgette & Carrot Noodles, 108
    Restorative Chicken Noodle Soup, 86–7

nut butters/creams
    Blueberry Almond Bread, 66–7
    Crispy Cauliflower Popcorn, 168–9
    Granola Fruit Bowl, 141
    Mocha Swirl Cheesecake, 150–1
    Raw Pad Thai with Courgette & Carrot Noodles, 108
    vegan, 153

nuts
    beneficial fats, 28
    butters, 28
    nut milks, 40
    and polyphenols, 30
    See also specific nuts

O

oats, 17
    Overnight Oats with Kiwi & Pomegranate, 84

oils
    olive oil. see olive oil
    as part of healthy diet, 28

oily fish, 24, 30
    See also mackerel; trout

olive oil, 39, 138, 169
    Lentil & Goat's Cheese Salad with Roasted Red Peppers, 111
    Poached Eggs with Wilted Kale, Tomato & Dukka, 82–3

olives, 30
    Braised Chicken with Green Olives
        & Preserved Lemon, 114–15
    Chicken & Artichoke Salad with
        Roasted Garlic & Herb Dressing,
        93
    Cumin-Spiced Halibut with Kale
        Salad, 132–3
omega-3 fats. See fats
onions, 19, 23, 24
    Asian-Spiced Lettuce Wraps, 94–5
    Broccoli & Watercress Cleanse, 92
    Chicken & Artichoke Salad with
        Roasted Garlic & Herb Dressing,
        93
    and FODMAPs, 17
    fructans, 20
    Pan-Fried Indian-Spiced Liver, 77
    Poached Eggs with Wilted Kale,
        Tomato & Dukka, 82–3
    Restorative Chicken Noodle Soup,
        86–7
    Spiced Omelette, 80–1
    Tempeh & Mushroom Bolognese,
        140
    See also red onions; shallots; spring
        onions
oranges/orange juice
    Citrus Mojito Kombucha, 58
    Fluffy Coconut Blinis with Spiced
        Fruit Compote, 74–5
    Paleo Carrot & Ginger Cake, 158–9
    Raw Mango, Turmeric & Cardamom
        Tart, 150
    Raw Orange Brownie Slices, 155
Overnight Oats with Kiwi &
    Pomegranate, 84

P
pak choi/bok choy
    Tamarind-Glazed Mackerel, 104–5
    Tofu Rice Bowl with Miso-Lemon
        Dressing, 139

Paleo bread, 113
    Paleo Carrot & Ginger Cake, 158–9
pancakes and blinis, Fluffy Coconut
    Blinis with Spiced Fruit Compote,
    74–5
Pan-Fried Indian-Spiced Liver, 77
Pan-Seared Venison with Blueberries &
    Broccoli Mash, 122–3
papaya, Tropical Fruit Platter with
    Sweet Ginger & Mint Dressing, 146–7
paprika
    Baked Chicken with Barbecue
        Sauce, 116–17
    Crispy Cauliflower Popcorn, 169
    Tempeh & Mushroom Bolognese,
        140
parsley
    Braised Chicken with Green Olives
        & Preserved Lemon, 114–15
    Lentil & Goat's Cheese Salad with
        Roasted Red Peppers, 111
    Pomegranate Lamb Tagine with
        Cauliflower Rice, 122–3
peanuts, Tofu Rice Bowl with Miso-
    Lemon Dressing, 139
pears, Green Gut Healer, 61
pecan nuts
    Apple & Plum Crisp, 152–3
    Breakfast Seed Bars, 69
    Mocha Swirl Cheesecake, 150–1
    Raw Orange Brownie Slices, 155
pectin, 20, 148
peppermint oil, 30
peppers, 24
    Asian-Spiced Lettuce Wraps, 94–5
    Chia, Flaxseed & Tomato Crackers,
        162–3
    Harissa Roasted Tofu Salad, 110
    Red Pepper and Chilli Vegan
        Mayonnaise, 39
    Vietnamese Prawn & Bacon Fried
        "Rice," 134–5
    See also red peppers

pesto, Hot-Smoked Trout with Pistachio
    Pesto Noodles, 102–3
phosphorus, 37, 44
Pickled Dill Cucumber, 51
pickles, 22, 50–5
pine nuts
    Mandarin Salad of Duck with Green
        Beans, 120
    Sicilian Tabbouleh with Cauliflower
        Rice, 109
pineapples
    Asian-Spiced Lettuce Wraps, 94–5
    Creamy Turmeric Kefir, 61
    Paleo Carrot & Ginger Cake, 158–9
    Tropical Fruit Platter with Sweet
        Ginger & Mint Dressing, 146–7
pistachio nuts, 28
    Hot-Smoked Trout with Pistachio
        Pesto Noodles, 102–3
pizza, Broccoli Pizza, 96–7
plant proteins, 28
plant-based diet, and your gut
    microbes, 9
plums
    Apple & Plum Crisp, 148–9
    Fluffy Coconut Blinis with Spiced
        Fruit Compote, 74–5
Poached Eggs with Wilted Kale, Tomato
    & Dukka, 82–3
polyols, 11, 13
polyphenols, 9, 17, 30, 113, 148, 159
polysaccharides, 124
pomegranate
    Cherry & Coconut Layered Parfait,
        144–5
    Lebanese Lamb Salad, 98–9
    Overnight Oats with Kiwi &
        Pomegranate, 84
    Pomegranate Lamb Tagine with
        Cauliflower Rice, 122–3
poppy seeds, Fennel & Poppy-Seed
    Crispbreads, 160–1
pork

Asian-Spiced Lettuce Wraps, 94–5
Southern-Spiced Pulled Pork with
  Sauerkraut, 119
  See also bacon
potatoes, prebiotics and, 17
poultry
  bone broth, 23, 37
  protein, 24
prawns/shrimps
  Asian Coconut Broth with Prawn
    Dumplings, 90–1
  Grilled Prawns with Turmeric Lemon
    Aioli, 106–7
  Vietnamese Prawn & Bacon Fried
    "Rice," 134–5
prebiotics, 9, 17, 23, 109, 138, 151
probiotics, 17, 20, 24, 138, 139
  for bloating, 21
  supplements, 20, 31
  yogurt for, 143
propionate, 9, 14
protein
  amino acids, 23
  milk/kefir, 140
  as part of healthy diet, 27–8
prunes, 20
psoriasis, 9
pumpkin, Pumpkin & Cinnamon Paleo
  Granola, 70
pumpkin seeds
  Chia, Flaxseed & Tomato Crackers,
    162–3
  Fennel & Poppy-Seed Crispbreads,
    160–1
Purple-Sprouting Broccoli & Beef Kelp
  Noodle Salad, 100

Q

quercetin, 24
quiches, Spinach, Tomato & Red
  Pepper Almond-Crusted Quiche,
  136–7

R

radishes, 22
  Lebanese Lamb Salad, 98–9
  Tofu Rice Bowl with Miso-Lemon
    Dressing, 139
  Turmeric-Infused Daikon, Red
    Radish & Ginger Pickle, 55
raisins, Raw Mango, Turmeric &
  Cardamom Tart, 150
ras el hanout, 123
Raw Mango, Turmeric & Cardamom
  Tart, 150
Raw Orange Brownie Slices, 151
Raw Pad Thai with Courgette & Carrot
  Noodles, 108
Red Cabbage and Beetroot Sauerkraut,
  53
red onions
  Chicken & Artichoke Salad with
    Roasted Garlic & Herb Dressing,
    93
  Cod with Mediterranean Herb
    Dressing, 128–9
  Korean Spiced Beef with Kimchi,
    124–5
  Lentil & Goat's Cheese Salad with
    Roasted Red Peppers, 111
  Lime-Marinated Salmon Salad with
    Fennel & Mango, 101
  Sicilian Tabbouleh with Cauliflower
    Rice, 109
  Turkey Meatballs with Roasted
    Tomato Chipotle Sauce, 118–19
red peppers
  Asian-Spiced Lettuce Wraps, 94–5
  Barbecue Kale Crisps, 169
  Chia, Flaxseed & Tomato Crackers,
    162–3
  Harissa Roasted Tofu Salad, 110
  Hot-Smoked Trout with Pistachio
    Pesto Noodles, 102–3
  Korean Spiced Beef with Kimchi,
    124–5

Lebanese Lamb Salad, 98–9
Lentil & Goat's Cheese Salad with
  Roasted Red Peppers, 111
Raw Pad Thai with Courgette &
  Carrot Noodles, 108
Red Pepper and Chilli Vegan
  Mayonnaise, 39
Restorative Chicken Noodle Soup,
  86–7
Spinach, Tomato & Red Pepper
  Almond-Crusted Quiche,
  136–7
Turkey Meatballs with Roasted
  Tomato Chipotle Sauce, 116–17
Vietnamese Prawn & Bacon Fried
  "Rice," 134–5
rice, 17
  Tofu Rice Bowl with Miso-Lemon
    Dressing, 139
Roasted Whole Salmon with Sweet Soy
  & Star Anise, 127
rocket/arugula
  Chicken & Artichoke Salad with
    Roasted Garlic & Herb Dressing,
    93
  Lime-Marinated Salmon Salad with
    Fennel & Mango, 101
  Mandarin Salad of Duck with Green
    Beans, 120
Rome IV Criteria, 5

S

saffron, Braised Chicken with Green
  Olives & Preserved Lemon, 115
salad
  Asian-Spiced Lettuce Wraps, 94–5
  Chicken & Artichoke Salad with
    Roasted Garlic & Herb Dressing,
    93
  Cumin-Spiced Halibut with Kale
    Salad, 132–3
  Grilled Prawns with Turmeric Lemon
    Aioli, 106–7

Lebanese Lamb Salad, 98–9
Lentil & Goat's Cheese Salad with
Roasted Red Peppers, 111
Lime Marinated Salmon Salad with
Fennel & Mango, 101
Mandarin Salad of Duck with Green
Beans, 120
Raw Pad Thai with Courgette &
Carrot Noodles, 108
salmon
Lime-Marinated Salmon Salad with
Fennel & Mango, 101
Roasted Whole Salmon with Sweet
Soy & Star Anise, 127
Smoked Salmon with Sweet Potato
Apple Röstis, 76–7
salsa, Vegan Mexican Taco Bowl, 136
sauerkraut, 22, 29, 52
Spiced Omelette, 80–1
Seeded Paleo Bread, 66
seeds
Barbecue Kale Crisps, 169
Breakfast Seed Bars, 69
butters, 28
Chia, Flaxseed & Tomato Crackers,
162–3
Fennel & Poppy-Seed Crispbreads,
160–1
omega-3, 30
Overnight Oats with Kiwi &
Pomegranate, 84
Poached Eggs with Wilted Kale,
Tomato & Dukka, 82–3
Pumpkin & Cinnamon Paleo
Granola, 70
Sunflower Seed & Mushroom
Falafels with Tahini Lemon
Dressing, 135
See also flaxseeds; sesame seeds
selenium, 98, 129
sesame seeds
Cumin-Spiced Halibut with Kale
Salad, 132–3

Fennel & Poppy-Seed Crispbreads,
160–1
shallots
Asian-Spiced Lettuce Wraps, 94–5
Baked Chicken with Barbecue
Sauce, 116–17
Beef & Liver Burgers with Wasabi
Mayo, 128
Braised Chicken with Green Olives
& Preserved Lemon, 113
Mandarin Salad of Duck with Green
Beans, 120
shiitake mushrooms
Korean Spiced Beef with Kimchi,
124–5
Mandarin Salad of Duck with Green
Beans, 120
Tofu Rice Bowl with Miso-Lemon
Dressing, 139
Vietnamese Prawn & Bacon Fried
"Rice," 134–5
short-chain fatty acids (SCFAs), 6–7,
8, 9, 11, 38
fibre and, 14
prebiotics and, 17
shrimps/prawns. See prawns/shrimps
Sicilian Tabbouleh with Cauliflower
Rice, 109
skin, and your gut microbes, 9
sleep, 18, 25, 26
slippery elm powder, 24, 61
small intestinal bacterial overgrowth
(SIBO), 7, 9, 20–1
small intestine, and coeliac disease, 10,
13
Smoked Salmon with Sweet Potato
Apple Röstis, 76–7
smoking, and your gut microbes, 9
smoothies, herbal, 24
soluble fibre, 11, 14
soups
Restorative Chicken Noodle Soup,
86–7

Spiced Roasted Beetroot & Apple
Soup, 88–9
Southern-Spiced Pulled Pork with
Sauerkraut, 119
soy sauce
Barbecue Kale Crisps, 169
Chia, Flaxseed & Tomato Crackers,
162–3
Cumin-Spiced Halibut with Kale
Salad, 132–3
Korean Spiced Beef with Kimchi,
124–5
Roasted Whole Salmon with Sweet
Soy & Star Anise, 127
Sunflower Seed & Mushroom
Falafels with Tahini Lemon
Dressing, 135
spaghetti, Tempeh & Mushroom
Bolognese, 140
Speedy Kimchi, 54
Spiced Omelette, 80–1
Spiced Roasted Beetroot & Apple Soup,
88–9
spices
Vietnamese Prawn & Bacon Fried
"Rice," 134–5
See also specific spices
spinach, 21
Asian Coconut Broth with Prawn
Dumplings, 90–1
Hot-Smoked Trout with Pistachio
Pesto Noodles, 102–3
Korean Spiced Beef with Kimchi,
124–5
Light Digestive Lemon Aid, 60
Raw Pad Thai with Courgette &
Carrot Noodles, 108
Spinach, Tomato & Red Pepper
Almond-Crusted Quiche, 136–7
Tofu Scramble, 85
spring onions
Asian Coconut Broth with Prawn
Dumplings, 90–1

spring onions (*continued*)
  Purple-Sprouting Broccoli & Beef Kelp Noodle Salad, 100
  Restorative Chicken Noodle Soup, 86–7
  Roasted Whole Salmon with Sweet Soy & Star Anise, 127
  Sicilian Tabbouleh with Cauliflower Rice, 109
  Spiced Omelette, 80–1
  Tofu Scramble, 85
star anise, Roasted Whole Salmon with Sweet Soy & Star Anise, 127
stock. *See* bone broth; vegetable stock
stomach acid, 7, 8, 22, 25
stress, 18, 19, 64
  and IBS, 6
  managing, 24–6
  and your gut microbes, 9
sugars
  coconut, 124, 133
  reducing, 22, 29
  Tamarind-Glazed Mackerel, 104
sumac powder, 98
Sunflower Seed & Mushroom Falafels with Tahini Lemon Dressing, 135
sunflower seeds
  Barbecue Kale Crisps, 169
  Fennel & Poppy-Seed Crispbreads, 160–1
supplements, 19, 21, 24, 26, 30–1
sweet potatoes, 30
  Harissa Roasted Tofu Salad, 110
  Smoked Salmon with Sweet Potato Apple Röstis, 76–7
sweeteners, 13, 20, 29
  See also sugars

T

Tabasco sauce, 126
tabbouleh, Sicilian Tabbouleh with Cauliflower Rice, 109
tagine, Pomegranate Lamb Tagine with

Cauliflower Rice, 122–3
tahini, Sunflower Seed & Mushroom Falafels with Tahini Lemon Dressing, 135
tamari soy sauce
  Baked Chicken with Barbecue Sauce, 116–17
  Barbecue Kale Crisps, 169
  Chia, Flaxseed & Tomato Crackers, 162–3
  Cumin-Spiced Halibut with Kale Salad, 132–3
  Mandarin Salad of Duck with Green Beans, 120
  Purple-Sprouting Broccoli & Beef Kelp Noodle Salad, 100
  Tempeh & Mushroom Bolognese, 140
  Tofu Rice Bowl with Miso-Lemon Dressing, 139
Tamarind-Glazed Mackerel, 104–5
tapioca flour
  Lemon Cream Sandwich Cookies, 156–7
  Spinach, Tomato & Red Pepper Almond-Crusted Quiche, 136–7
tarts, Raw Mango, Turmeric & Cardamom Tart, 150
tea, 19, 21, 25
  See also green tea
Tempeh & Mushroom Bolognese, 140
tofu, 28, 103
  Harissa Roasted Tofu Salad, 110
  Raw Orange Brownie Slices, 151
  Tofu Rice Bowl with Miso-Lemon Dressing, 139
  Tofu Scramble, 85
tomatoes
  Baked Chicken with Barbecue Sauce, 116–17
  Chicken & Artichoke Salad with Roasted Garlic & Herb Dressing, 93

Chipotle Avocado Cream Spread, 168
Cumin-Spiced Halibut with Kale Salad, 132–3
Harissa Roasted Tofu Salad, 110
Hot-Smoked Trout with Pistachio Pesto Noodles, 102–3
Lebanese Lamb Salad, 98–9
Pan-Fried Indian-Spiced Liver, 77
Poached Eggs with Wilted Kale, Tomato & Dukka, 82–3
Pomegranate Lamb Tagine with Cauliflower Rice, 122–3
Sicilian Tabbouleh with Cauliflower Rice, 109
Spinach, Tomato & Red Pepper Almond-Crusted Quiche, 136–7
Tempeh & Mushroom Bolognese, 140
Tofu Scramble, 85
Turkey Meatballs with Roasted Tomato Chipotle Sauce, 116–17
Vegan Mexican Taco Bowl, 134
tomatoes, sun-dried
  Barbecue Kale Crisps, 169
  Chia, Flaxseed & Tomato Crackers, 162–3
  Sunflower Seed & Mushroom Falafels with Tahini Lemon Dressing, 135
Tropical Fruit Platter with Sweet Ginger & Mint Dressing, 146–7
trout, Hot-Smoked Trout with Pistachio Pesto Noodles, 102–3
Turkey Meatballs with Roasted Tomato Chipotle Sauce, 118–19
turmeric, 24
  Asian Coconut Broth with Prawn Dumplings, 90–1
  Braised Chicken with Green Olives & Preserved Lemon, 112–13
  Creamy Turmeric Kefir, 61

Crispy Cauliflower Popcorn, 169
Grilled Prawns with Turmeric Lemon
    Aioli, 106–7
Raw Mango, Turmeric & Cardamom
    Tart, 150
Spiced Omelette, 80–1
supplements, 31
Turmeric-Infused Daikon, Red
    Radish & Ginger Pickle, 55

U
urinary issues, and IBS, 5

V
vagus nerve, 8
Vegan Mexican Taco Bowl, 134
Vegan Nut Cream, 48
veganism, and FODMAPs, 11–12
vegetable stock
    Broccoli & Watercress Cleanse, 92
    Spiced Roasted Beetroot & Apple
        Soup, 88–9
vegetables, 28
    balance and variety, 30
    brassicas, 169
    Broccoli Pizza, 96–7
    cruciferous, 23
    See also specific types of vegetable
venison, Pan-Seared Venison with
    Blueberries & Broccoli Mash, 122–3
Vietnamese Prawn & Bacon Fried
    "Rice," 134–5
vinegar, 21
    apple cider, 37, 119, 135
    in herb dressings, 93
    rice wine, 127, 139

See also balsamic vinegar
vitamins, 38, 165–6
    B vitamins, 39, 44, 94, 98, 120, 164
    fat-soluble, deficiencies in, 7
    for repairing the gut, 23
    vitamin A, 126, 136
    vitamin C, 114
    vitamin D, 104, 124, 129, 135
    vitamin E, 91, 164

W
waffles, Buttermilk Waffles with Berries,
    74
walnuts
    Lentil & Goat's Cheese Salad with
        Roasted Red Peppers, 111
    Paleo Carrot & Ginger Cake, 158–9
    Pumpkin & Cinnamon Paleo
        Granola, 70
    Vegan Mexican Taco Bowl, 134
wasabi, 22
    Beef & Liver Burgers with Wasabi
        Mayo, 128
water, drinking, 29
water kefir, 45
    Fruity Gummy Sweets, 159
watercress, Broccoli & Watercress
    Cleanse, 92
wellbeing. See mood/wellbeing
wheat, 14, 21, 23
wholegrains, 14
Worcestershire sauce, 126

X
xylitol, 13, 101, 104, 153, 154

Y
yeast flakes
    Barbecue Kale Crisps, 169
    Broccoli Pizza, 96–7
    Crispy Cauliflower Popcorn, 169
    Cumin-Spiced Halibut with Kale
        Salad, 132–3
    Sunflower Seed & Mushroom
        Falafels with Tahini Lemon
        Dressing, 135
    Tempeh & Mushroom Bolognese,
        140
    Tofu Rice Bowl with Miso-Lemon
        Dressing, 139
yeasts, 29, 44
yoga, 25
yogurt, 20, 29, 46–7
    Cherry & Coconut Layered Parfait,
        144–5
    Chipotle Avocado Cream Spread, 167
    Hot-Smoked Trout with Pistachio
        Pesto Noodles, 102–3
    Overnight Oats with Kiwi &
        Pomegranate, 84
    Smoked Salmon with Sweet Potato
        Apple Röstis, 76–7
    Tropical Fruit Platter with Sweet
        Ginger & Mint Dressing, 146–7

Z
zinc, 22, 39, 94, 98, 117, 148
    Pumpkin & Cinnamon Paleo
        Granola, 70
    Southern-Spiced Pulled Pork with
        Sauerkraut, 119
    Tofu Scramble, 85

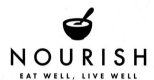

NOURISH

EAT WELL, LIVE WELL

Here at Nourish we're all about wellbeing through food and drink – irresistible dishes with a serious good-for-you factor. If you want to eat and drink delicious things that set you up for the day, suit any special diets, keep you healthy and make the most of the ingredients you have, we've got some great ideas to share with you. Come over to our blog for wholesome recipes and fresh inspiration – nourishbooks.com